DISEASE GUIDE BOOK

Diseases & Conditions That Affect Human Body

DR. KRIS DAVIS

Table of contents

INTRODUCTION

In this comprehensive guidebook on diseases, I delve into the intricate **details** of various health conditions. From exploring and discussing preventive measures, effective cures, and **advanced** detection techniques, this book aims to equip readers with a thorough understanding of diverse ailments. As you embark on this journey through the pages, my hope is that this guide serves as a **valuable** and **insightful** resource for everyone seeking knowledge on maintaining and improving health.

Chapter 1

Cardiovascular conditions

Cardiovascular conditions refer to a group of disorders that affect the heart and blood vessels. The cardiovascular system is crucial for maintaining overall health, as it is responsible for pumping blood throughout the body, delivering oxygen and nutrients to various tissues and organs. Here are some common cardiovascular conditions:

•**Coronary Artery Disease (CAD)**: This condition occurs when the blood vessels that supply the heart muscle with oxygen and nutrients (coronary arteries) become narrowed or blocked due to the buildup of plaque. Reduced blood flow to the heart can lead to chest pain (angina) or result in a heart attack.

•**Hypertension (High Blood Pressure)**: High blood pressure occurs when the force of blood against the walls of the arteries is consistently too high. Over time, untreated hypertension can lead to serious cardiovascular problems, including heart disease, stroke, and heart failure.

•**Heart Failure**: This is a condition where the heart is unable to pump blood effectively, leading to insufficient blood supply to meet the body's needs. Heart failure can result from various cardiovascular conditions, such as CAD, hypertension, or a previous heart attack.

•**Arrhythmias**: Arrhythmias are abnormalities in the heart's rhythm or heartbeat. This can manifest as an irregular, too fast, or too slow heartbeat. Arrhythmias can be harmless or serious, affecting the heart's ability to pump blood effectively.

•**Valvular Heart Disease**: This condition involves damage or defects in the heart valves, which can affect blood flow within the heart. It may be due to conditions like infections, congenital defects, or age-related changes.

•**Stroke**: While not a heart condition per se, strokes are often related to cardiovascular health. A stroke occurs when there is a disruption of blood flow to the brain, either due to a blocked artery (ischemic stroke) or a ruptured blood vessel (hemorrhagic stroke).

Preventive measures for cardiovascular conditions include maintaining a healthy lifestyle with regular exercise, a balanced diet, avoiding tobacco, and managing stress. Early detection and management of risk factors, such as high blood pressure and high cholesterol, are crucial for preventing the development of cardiovascular diseases. Regular medical check-ups and consultations with healthcare professionals are important for monitoring and addressing potential cardiovascular issues.

Coronary Artery Disease (CAD)

Coronary Artery Disease (CAD) is a common and serious cardiovascular condition that primarily affects the coronary arteries, the blood vessels responsible for supplying oxygen and nutrients to the heart muscle. CAD is often referred to as atherosclerosis or coronary heart disease.

1. **Atherosclerosis**:

Cause: The primary cause of CAD is atherosclerosis, a condition characterized by the buildup of fatty deposits, cholesterol, calcium, and other substances, collectively known as plaque, on the inner walls of the coronary arteries.

Process: Over time, this plaque can harden and narrow the arteries, reducing blood flow to the heart muscle. In some cases, the plaque may rupture, leading to the formation of blood clots that can further block the arteries.

Risk Factors

Modifiable Factors: Certain lifestyle factors contribute to the development of CAD, including smoking, high blood pressure, high cholesterol levels, obesity, lack of physical activity, and an unhealthy diet high in saturated and trans fats.
Non-modifiable Factors: Age, gender (men are generally at higher risk), family history, and genetic factors also play a role in CAD risk.

Symptoms

CAD may progress without noticeable symptoms for a long time. However, as the arteries narrow, symptoms may develop, including:
•Chest pain or discomfort (angina), often triggered by physical exertion or emotional stress.
•Shortness of breath.
•Fatigue.
•Sweating.
•Nausea.

Complications

•Myocardial Infarction (Heart Attack): If a coronary artery becomes completely blocked, it can lead to a heart attack. The lack of blood flow can cause damage or death to part of the heart muscle.

•Chronic Heart Failure: CAD can eventually weaken the heart, leading to heart failure, where the heart is unable to pump blood effectively to meet the body's needs.

•Arrhythmias: CAD increases the risk of irregular heartbeats (arrhythmias) due to the compromised blood supply to the heart.

Diagnosis

CAD can be diagnosed through various tests, including electrocardiograms (ECG or EKG), stress tests, coronary angiography, CT scans, and blood tests to assess cholesterol levels.

Treatment

Medications: Medications may be prescribed to manage risk factors, including cholesterol-lowering drugs, blood pressure medications, and antiplatelet medications to prevent blood clot formation.

Procedures: In more severe cases, interventions such as angioplasty and stent placement or coronary artery bypass grafting (CABG) may be recommended to improve blood flow to the heart.

Prevention and early intervention are key in managing CAD. Regular medical check-ups, monitoring risk factors, and seeking prompt medical attention for symptoms are important components of CAD management.

<u>Hypertension (High Blood Pressure)</u>

Hypertension, commonly known as high blood pressure, is a condition where the force of the blood against the walls of the arteries is consistently too high. Blood pressure is the measurement of the force exerted by blood against the walls of the arteries as the heart pumps it around the body. It is measured in millimeters of mercury (mmHg) and is recorded as two numbers: systolic pressure over diastolic pressure.

Categories of Blood Pressure

•Normal: Blood pressure is considered normal when it is around 120/80 mmHg.
Hypertension: Hypertension is typically defined as having a blood pressure consistently higher than 130/80 mmHg. It is further categorized into stages:
•Stage 1 Hypertension: 130-139/80-89 mmHg
•Stage 2 Hypertension: 140/90 mmHg or higher

Causes and Risk Factors

•Primary (Essential) Hypertension: The majority of cases (about 90-95%) fall into this category, and the exact cause is often unknown. It tends to develop gradually over many years.

•Secondary Hypertension: This form is caused by an underlying condition, such as kidney disease, hormonal disorders, or certain medications.

Risk Factors Include:

•Age (Risk increases with age)
•Family history
•Race (African Americans tend to develop
•hypertension more often and at an earlier age)
•Obesity
•Lack of physical activity
•High salt intake
•Excessive alcohol consumption
•Chronic kidney disease
•Sleep apnea

Symptoms

Hypertension is often called the "silent killer" because it may not cause noticeable symptoms for years. Many people with high blood pressure are unaware of their condition until it is detected during a routine checkup.

In severe cases, symptoms may include headaches, shortness of breath, nosebleeds, or dizziness.

Complications

•Heart Disease: Hypertension is a major risk factor for coronary artery disease, heart attack, and heart failure.

•Stroke: High blood pressure can damage blood vessels in the brain, leading to strokes.

Kidney Disease: Prolonged hypertension can damage the kidneys, reducing their ability to function properly.

•Eye Damage: Hypertension can affect the blood vessels in the eyes, potentially leading to vision problems or even blindness.

Diagnosis

Blood pressure is measured using a sphygmomanometer. A reading above the normal range on multiple occasions is required for a diagnosis of hypertension.

Ambulatory blood pressure monitoring (ABPM) or home blood pressure monitoring may be recommended to confirm the diagnosis.

Treatment

Lifestyle Changes: These include adopting a healthy diet (such as the DASH diet rich in fruits, vegetables, and low-fat dairy products), regular exercise, weight management, limiting alcohol intake, and reducing sodium consumption.

Medications: Antihypertensive medications may be prescribed when lifestyle changes alone are insufficient. These medications work to lower blood pressure and may include diuretics, beta-blockers, ACE inhibitors, angiotensin II receptor blockers (ARBs), calcium channel blockers, and others.

Hypertension is a chronic condition that requires ongoing management. Regular monitoring, adherence to prescribed medications, and a commitment to a healthy lifestyle are crucial in controlling blood pressure and reducing the risk of complications. It's important for individuals to work closely with healthcare professionals to develop and maintain an effective treatment plan.

Heart Failure

Heart failure is a chronic condition in which the heart is unable to pump blood effectively to meet the body's demands. It doesn't mean that the heart has stopped working, but rather that it is not pumping blood as well as it should. Heart failure can affect the left side, the right side, or both sides of the heart.

Types of Heart Failure

Left-Sided Heart Failure:

•Systolic Heart Failure: The left ventricle loses its ability to contract effectively, reducing the amount of blood pumped out with each heartbeat.
•Diastolic Heart Failure: The left ventricle loses its ability to relax properly, preventing it from filling with enough blood between beats.
•Right-Sided Heart Failure: The right ventricle loses its ability to pump blood to the lungs effectively, leading to fluid buildup in the body's extremities.

Causes

•Coronary Artery Disease (CAD): A common cause that can weaken the heart muscle.
•Myocardial Infarction (Heart Attack): Damage to the heart muscle from a heart attack can lead to heart failure.
•Hypertension (High Blood Pressure): Chronic high blood pressure forces the heart to work harder, leading to heart muscle damage.
•Cardiomyopathy: Diseases that affect the heart muscle directly can lead to heart failure.
•Valvular Heart Diseases: Disorders of the heart valves can contribute to heart failure.

Symptoms

Symptoms can vary, but common ones include:
Shortness of breath, especially during exertion or when lying down.
Persistent coughing or wheezing.
Fluid retention, leading to swelling in the legs, ankles, and abdomen.
•Fatigue and weakness.
•Rapid or irregular heartbeat.
•Reduced ability to exercise.

Diagnosis

•Physical Examination: Healthcare professionals may look for signs of fluid retention, listen for abnormal heart sounds, and assess overall health.
•Imaging Tests: Echocardiograms, chest X-rays, and other imaging tests can provide detailed information about the structure and function of the heart.
•Blood Tests: These may be conducted to check for markers of heart failure and other related conditions.

Treatment

•Lifestyle Changes: Patients are often advised to make changes such as adopting a low-sodium diet, managing fluid intake, quitting smoking, and engaging in regular exercise.

Medications: Various medications may be prescribed to manage symptoms and improve heart function. These may include diuretics, ACE inhibitors, beta-blockers, and others.

•Implantable Devices: Devices such as pacemakers or defibrillators may be recommended in certain cases.

•Surgery: In some instances, heart surgery or procedures like heart valve repair or heart transplant may be considered.

Management and Prognosis

Heart failure is a chronic condition that requires ongoing management to control symptoms and improve quality of life.

While heart failure is a serious condition, advances in medical treatments have improved outcomes, and many people with heart failure can lead fulfilling lives with proper management.

It's crucial for individuals with heart failure to work closely with healthcare professionals to develop and follow a comprehensive treatment plan tailored to their specific needs. Regular medical check-ups and monitoring are essential to adjust treatment as needed and to manage the condition effectively.

Arrhythmias

Arrhythmias refer to abnormal heart rhythms or irregular heartbeats. The heart's normal rhythm is coordinated by electrical signals that regulate the timing of each heartbeat. When these electrical signals are disrupted or irregular, it can lead to various types of arrhythmias.

Types of Arrhythmias

•Atrial Fibrillation (AFib): The atria (upper chambers of the heart) quiver instead of contracting effectively, leading to an irregular and often rapid heartbeat.
•Atrial Flutter: Similar to AFib, but the atria beat in a more organized, regular pattern.
Supraventricular Tachycardia (SVT): Episodes of rapid heart rate originating above the heart's ventricles.
•Ventricular Tachycardia: Rapid heart rate originating in the heart's lower chambers (ventricles).
Ventricular Fibrillation: Rapid, chaotic heartbeat that can be life-threatening and requires immediate medical attention.

Causes

•Coronary Artery Disease (CAD): Reduced blood flow to the heart muscle can disrupt the heart's electrical system.

•Heart Attack: Damage to the heart muscle can disrupt the normal electrical pathways.

•High Blood Pressure: Chronic high blood pressure can strain the heart and lead to arrhythmias.

•Heart Valve Disorders: Abnormalities in the heart valves can disrupt blood flow and trigger arrhythmias.

•Heart Failure: Weakened heart muscles may result in irregular heart rhythms.

•Congenital Heart Defects: Structural abnormalities present at birth can affect the heart's electrical system.

Symptoms

Symptoms can vary widely depending on the type and severity of the arrhythmia. Common symptoms include:

•Palpitations (feeling of rapid, fluttering, or pounding heartbeat).

•Chest discomfort or pain.

•Dizziness or lightheadedness.

•Fainting (syncope).

•Shortness of breath.

•Fatigue.

Diagnosis

Electrocardiogram (ECG or EKG): A primary diagnostic tool that records the heart's electrical activity.

Holter Monitor: A portable ECG device worn for a continuous period (usually 24 to 48 hours) to monitor heart activity over time.

Event Monitor: Similar to a Holter monitor but used for shorter periods to record specific events or symptoms.

Electrophysiology (EP) Study: Invasive testing to study the heart's electrical system and locate the source of the arrhythmia.

Treatment

•Medications: Antiarrhythmic drugs may be prescribed to regulate the heart's rhythm.

•Cardioversion: A controlled electric shock to restore a normal heart rhythm.

•Catheter Ablation: A minimally invasive procedure to destroy abnormal heart tissue causing the arrhythmia.

•Implantable Devices: Pacemakers can help regulate slow heart rhythms, while implantable cardioverter-defibrillators (ICDs) can monitor and treat life-threatening arrhythmias.

Lifestyle Changes: These may include avoiding stimulants like caffeine, managing stress, and making dietary changes.

Prognosis

The prognosis for individuals with arrhythmias varies depending on the type and severity of the condition.

Many people with arrhythmias can manage their condition effectively with medical treatments and lifestyle changes.

♦It's important for individuals experiencing symptoms of arrhythmias to seek medical attention for a proper diagnosis and appropriate management. Treatment plans are often tailored to the specific type of arrhythmia and the individual's overall health. Regular follow-up with healthcare professionals is crucial for ongoing monitoring and adjustment of treatment as needed.

Valvular Heart Disease

Valvular heart disease refers to conditions that affect one or more of the heart's valves. The heart has four valves — the mitral valve, tricuspid valve, aortic valve, and pulmonary valve — which play a crucial role in ensuring the unidirectional flow of blood through the heart. Valvular heart disease can involve the malfunction, stenosis (narrowing), or regurgitation (leakage) of these valves.

Types of Valvular Heart Disease:

•Mitral Valve Prolapse (MVP): The mitral valve leaflets bulge back into the left atrium during the heart's contraction.
•Aortic Stenosis: Narrowing of the aortic valve, reducing the flow of blood from the left ventricle to the aorta.
•Mitral Stenosis: Narrowing of the mitral valve, impeding blood flow from the left atrium to the left ventricle.
•Aortic Regurgitation: The aortic valve doesn't close properly, allowing blood to flow back into the left ventricle.
•Mitral Regurgitation: The mitral valve doesn't close properly, allowing blood to flow back into the left atrium.
•Tricuspid Regurgitation: The tricuspid valve doesn't close properly, allowing blood to flow back into the right atrium.
•Tricuspid Stenosis: Narrowing of the tricuspid valve, hindering blood flow from the right atrium to the right ventricle.

•Pulmonary Regurgitation: The pulmonary valve doesn't close properly, allowing blood to flow back into the right ventricle.

Causes

•Congenital Heart Defects: Some individuals are born with valve abnormalities.

•Rheumatic Fever: A complication of untreated streptococcal infections can cause damage to heart valves.

•Age-Related Changes: Wear and tear on heart valves over time can lead to valvular heart disease.

Infective Endocarditis: Infection of the heart valves can cause damage.

•Calcification: Calcium deposits on the valves can cause them to become stiff and narrowed.

Symptoms

•Cardiac Catheterization: Invasive testing using a catheter to evaluate blood flow and pressure within the heart.

Treatment

•Medications: Depending on the type of valvular heart disease, medications may be prescribed to manage symptoms or prevent complications.

•Valve Repair or Replacement: In some cases, damaged valves may be surgically repaired or replaced.

•Balloon Valvuloplasty: A catheter with a balloon is used to widen a narrowed valve.
•Antibiotics: In cases of infective endocarditis, antibiotics may be prescribed to treat the infection.

Prognosis

The prognosis for valvular heart disease depends on factors such as the type and severity of the condition, the presence of symptoms, and how well it responds to treatment.
With appropriate management, many people with valvular heart disease can lead normal, active lives.
Regular follow-up with healthcare professionals is essential for monitoring the progression of valvular heart disease and adjusting the treatment plan as needed. In some cases, individuals may need lifelong monitoring and management.

Stroke

A stroke, also known as a cerebrovascular accident (CVA), is a medical emergency that occurs when there is a sudden disruption of blood flow to the brain, leading to damage to brain cells. The lack of blood flow may result from a blocked artery (ischemic stroke) or the rupture of a blood vessel (hemorrhagic stroke). Strokes can cause a range of symptoms and complications, and prompt medical attention is crucial to minimize brain damage and improve outcomes.

Types of Strokes

•Ischemic Stroke: This is the most common type, accounting for about 87% of all strokes. It occurs when a blood clot or plaque blocks a blood vessel, reducing or cutting off blood flow to a part of the brain.
•Hemorrhagic Stroke: This type results from the rupture of a blood vessel in the brain, leading to bleeding into the surrounding tissues.

Causes and Risk Factors

Ischemic Stroke: Common causes include atherosclerosis (narrowing of the arteries due to plaque buildup), blood clots, and embolisms (traveling blood clots).
Hemorrhagic Stroke: Causes include high blood pressure (hypertension), aneurysms (weakened blood vessel walls), arteriovenous malformations

(abnormal tangles of blood vessels), and bleeding disorders.

Risk Factors: Common risk factors for strokes include age, gender (men have a slightly higher risk), high blood pressure, smoking, diabetes, high cholesterol, atrial fibrillation, family history, and previous history of stroke or transient ischemic attack (TIA).

Symptoms

The symptoms of a stroke can vary depending on the type and location of the brain affected. Common symptoms include:

Sudden numbness or weakness in the face, arm, or leg, especially on one side of the body.

Sudden confusion, trouble speaking, or difficulty understanding speech.

Sudden trouble seeing in one or both eyes.

Sudden severe headache with no apparent cause.

Diagnosis

Clinical Assessment: Healthcare professionals will conduct a physical examination and assess the patient's symptoms.

Imaging Tests: CT (computed tomography) scans or MRI (magnetic resonance imaging) scans are used to visualize the brain and identify the type and location of the stroke.

Blood Tests: These may be conducted to check for conditions that may contribute to stroke risk.

Treatment

Ischemic Stroke: Treatment often involves restoring blood flow to the brain. This may be achieved through the administration of clot-busting medications (thrombolytics) or mechanical clot retrieval procedures.

Hemorrhagic Stroke: Treatment focuses on controlling bleeding, reducing pressure in the brain, and addressing the underlying cause.

Rehabilitation: Following the acute phase, stroke survivors often require rehabilitation to regain lost skills and improve overall function.

Complications

Strokes can lead to various complications, including paralysis, cognitive impairments, difficulty speaking or swallowing, emotional changes, and increased risk of future strokes.

Prevention

Managing risk factors through lifestyle changes, such as maintaining a healthy diet, exercising regularly, quitting smoking, managing stress, and controlling chronic conditions like high blood pressure and diabetes, can help reduce the risk of stroke.

♦Strokes are medical emergencies, and rapid intervention is critical for minimizing brain damage. Recognizing the symptoms of a stroke and seeking immediate medical attention can significantly improve outcomes. Following a stroke, ongoing medical care, rehabilitation, and lifestyle changes are important for recovery and preventing future events.

Chapter 2

Respiratory conditions

Respiratory conditions refer to a variety of disorders that affect the respiratory system, which includes the organs and structures involved in breathing. The respiratory system's primary function is to facilitate the exchange of oxygen and carbon dioxide between the body and the external environment. Respiratory conditions can affect any part of this system, including the nose, throat, trachea, bronchi, and lungs.

Common respiratory conditions are:

Asthma:

Asthma is a chronic inflammatory condition that affects the airways. It can cause wheezing, shortness of breath, chest tightness, and coughing. Asthma symptoms can be triggered by various factors such as allergens, exercise, or exposure to irritants.

Chronic Obstructive Pulmonary Disease (COPD):

COPD is a progressive lung disease that includes chronic bronchitis and emphysema. It is often associated with long-term exposure to irritating gasses or particulate matter, typically from cigarette smoke. Symptoms include difficulty breathing, coughing, and excess mucus production.

Pneumonia:

Pneumonia is an infection that inflames the air sacs in one or both lungs. It can be caused by bacteria, viruses, or fungi. Symptoms include fever, cough, chest pain, and difficulty breathing. Pneumonia can range from mild to severe and may require medical intervention.

Cystic Fibrosis:

Cystic fibrosis is a genetic disorder that primarily affects the respiratory and digestive systems. It leads to the production of thick, sticky mucus that can clog the airways, making breathing difficult and increasing the risk of respiratory infections.

Obstructive Sleep Apnea (OSA):

OSA is a sleep disorder in which a person's airway becomes partially or completely blocked during sleep, leading to pauses in breathing. This can result in loud snoring, disrupted sleep, and daytime fatigue. OSA is often associated with other health conditions, including obesity.

Lung Cancer:

Lung cancer occurs when abnormal cells divide and grow uncontrollably in the lungs. It is often associated with smoking but can also occur in non-smokers. Symptoms may include persistent cough, chest pain, weight loss, and difficulty breathing.

It's crucial to note that the severity and treatment of respiratory conditions vary widely. Some conditions are chronic and require long-term management, while others may be acute and resolve with appropriate medical care. Early diagnosis and intervention are essential for improving outcomes in many respiratory conditions. If you or someone you know is experiencing respiratory symptoms, seeking medical advice is important for proper evaluation and treatment.

Asthma

Asthma is a chronic inflammatory condition that affects the airways, the tubes that carry air in and out of the lungs. In individuals with asthma, the airways are sensitive and tend to react strongly to certain triggers, causing various symptoms.

Causes and Triggers

Inflammation: Asthma involves chronic inflammation of the airways. This inflammation makes the airways more sensitive to various triggers.

Bronchoconstriction: When exposed to triggers, the muscles around the airways tighten (bronchoconstriction), and the airway lining swells, leading to a narrowing of the air passages.

Excessive Mucus Production: In response to triggers, the airways may produce excess mucus, further contributing to airway obstruction.

Common Triggers

Allergens: Common allergens that can trigger asthma include pollen, mold spores, pet dander, dust mites, and cockroach droppings.

Irritants: Exposure to irritants such as tobacco smoke, air pollution, strong odors, and chemical fumes can provoke asthma symptoms.

Respiratory Infections: Viral infections, particularly respiratory infections like the common cold, can exacerbate asthma symptoms.

Exercise: Physical activity can trigger asthma symptoms in some individuals, a condition known as exercise-induced bronchoconstriction.

Cold Air or Weather Changes: Exposure to cold air or sudden weather changes can provoke asthma symptoms.

Emotional Factors: Stress and strong emotions can sometimes trigger asthma symptoms.

Symptoms

Wheezing: A whistling or squeaky sound when breathing, particularly during exhalation.

Shortness of Breath: Difficulty breathing or feeling out of breath.

Coughing: Persistent coughing, especially at night or early in the morning.

Chest Tightness: A sensation of tightness or pressure in the chest.

Diagnosis

Medical History and Physical Examination: A doctor will inquire about symptoms, triggers, and family history and conduct a physical examination.

Lung Function Tests: Spirometry is a common test that measures how much air you can breathe out and how quickly. It helps in assessing airflow obstruction.

Peak Flow Measurements: A peak flow meter is a handheld device that measures the force of air during exhalation.

Treatment

Bronchodilators: These medications relax the muscles around the airways, opening them up and making it easier to breathe. Short-acting bronchodilators provide quick relief during an asthma attack.

Anti-Inflammatory Medications: Inhaled corticosteroids and other anti-inflammatory drugs help control chronic inflammation and prevent asthma symptoms.

Long-Term Control Medications: For individuals with persistent asthma, long-term control medications are often prescribed to manage symptoms and prevent exacerbations.

Allergen and Trigger Management: Identifying and avoiding asthma triggers is an essential part of managing the condition.

Lifestyle Modifications: Adopting a healthy lifestyle, including regular exercise and maintaining a smoke-free environment, can contribute to overall asthma management.

Education and Asthma Action Plan: Patients are often provided with an asthma action plan, which outlines steps to take based on symptoms and peak flow measurements.

♦It's important for individuals with asthma to work closely with healthcare professionals to develop a personalized asthma management plan. Regular follow-ups and adjustments to the treatment plan are often necessary to ensure optimal asthma control and quality of life.

Chronic Obstructive Pulmonary Disease (COPD)

Chronic Obstructive Pulmonary Disease (COPD) is a progressive lung disease characterized by persistent respiratory symptoms and airflow limitation. The term COPD encompasses two main conditions: **chronic bronchitis and emphysema**. Both conditions contribute to the obstruction of airflow and make breathing difficult.

1. **Chronic Bronchitis**:
Definition: Chronic bronchitis involves inflammation and irritation of the bronchial tubes (airways) leading to increased mucus production.
Symptoms: Persistent cough with sputum production, shortness of breath, and frequent respiratory infections.
Pathophysiology: Inflammation of the bronchial tubes leads to the narrowing of airways, increased mucus production, and compromised airflow.

2. **Emphysema**:
Definition: Emphysema is characterized by the destruction of the air sacs (alveoli) in the lungs, reducing their elasticity.
Symptoms: Shortness of breath, especially with physical activity, and a feeling of not getting enough air.
Pathophysiology: Damage to the alveoli reduces the surface area available for oxygen exchange, leading to impaired airflow and decreased oxygenation of the blood.

Causes and Risk Factors

Smoking: The primary cause of COPD is long-term exposure to irritating gases or particulate matter, most commonly from cigarette smoke.

Occupational Exposures: Prolonged exposure to workplace pollutants such as dust, chemicals, and fumes can contribute to COPD.
Air Pollution: Long-term exposure to indoor and outdoor air pollution can increase the risk of developing COPD.

Genetic Factors: Some individuals may have a genetic predisposition to COPD, especially if they have a deficiency in a protein called alpha-1 antitrypsin.

Symptoms

•**Chronic Cough**: A persistent cough that may produce mucus.
•**Shortness of Breath**: Gradual development of breathlessness, initially during physical exertion and later even at rest.
•**Wheezing**: A whistling or squeaky sound when breathing.
•**Chest Tightness**: A feeling of constriction or pressure in the chest.

Diagnosis

Medical History and Physical Examination: The doctor will inquire about symptoms, risk factors, and conduct a physical examination.

Lung Function Tests: Spirometry measures the amount and speed of air that can be inhaled and exhaled, helping assess airflow limitation.

Imaging Studies: Chest X-rays and CT scans may be used to visualize the lungs and assess for structural changes.

Blood Tests: Blood tests may be conducted to rule out other conditions and assess oxygen levels.

Treatment

Smoking Cessation: The most important intervention is to stop smoking, as it can slow the progression of COPD.

Medications

Bronchodilators: These medications help relax the muscles around the airways, improving airflow.

Inhaled Corticosteroids: These reduce inflammation in the airways.

Phosphodiesterase-4 Inhibitors: These can reduce inflammation and relax the airways.

Pulmonary Rehabilitation: A comprehensive program involving exercise training, education, and support to improve quality of life.

Oxygen Therapy: For individuals with severe COPD, supplemental oxygen may be prescribed to improve oxygen levels.

Surgery: In advanced cases, lung volume reduction surgery or lung transplantation may be considered.

Management and Prognosis

COPD is a chronic condition that requires ongoing management. Lifestyle modifications, regular monitoring, and prompt treatment of exacerbations are crucial. Although COPD is not curable, proper management can significantly improve symptoms and slow down disease progression.

♦Early diagnosis and intervention, along with a collaborative approach involving healthcare professionals, can help individuals with COPD lead fulfilling lives despite the challenges posed by the condition.

Pneumonia

Pneumonia is an inflammatory condition of the lung affecting the air sacs, or alveoli, and can be caused by various infectious agents such as bacteria, viruses, fungi, or other microorganisms. It is characterized by inflammation, consolidation (filling with fluid or pus), and sometimes the formation of abscesses in the lungs. Pneumonia can range from mild to severe and can affect one or both lungs.

Causes of Pneumonia

Bacterial Pneumonia: Common bacteria responsible for pneumonia include Streptococcus pneumoniae, Haemophilus influenzae, and Staphylococcus aureus.

Viral Pneumonia: Viruses such as influenza (flu), respiratory syncytial virus (RSV), and adenovirus can cause pneumonia.

Mycoplasma Pneumonia: A type of atypical pneumonia caused by the bacterium Mycoplasma pneumoniae.

Fungal Pneumonia: Fungi like Pneumocystis jirovecii can cause pneumonia, especially in individuals with weakened immune systems.

Aspiration Pneumonia: This occurs when foreign substances, such as food, liquids, or vomit, are inhaled into the lungs, leading to infection.

Symptoms

Cough: May produce phlegm that can be green, yellow, or bloody.

Fever: Often accompanied by chills.

Shortness of Breath: Difficulty breathing, especially during physical activity.

Chest Pain: Sharp or stabbing pain, particularly during deep breaths or coughing.

Fatigue: Feeling unusually tired or weak.

Confusion: Particularly in older adults or those with weakened immune systems.

Diagnosis

Medical History and Physical Examination: The doctor will inquire about symptoms, medical history, and conduct a physical examination.

Chest X-ray: A common imaging test used to visualize the .lungs and identify areas of consolidation.

Blood Tests: To assess the severity of the infection and identify the causative agent.

Sputum Culture: If possible, a sample of sputum may be collected and analyzed to identify the specific microorganism causing the infection.

Treatment

Antibiotics: If the pneumonia is bacterial, antibiotics are prescribed to target the specific bacteria causing the infection.

Antiviral Medications: For viral pneumonia, antiviral drugs may be used to treat the underlying viral infection.

Antifungal Medications: Fungal pneumonia is treated with antifungal drugs.

Symptomatic Relief: Medications to reduce fever, relieve pain, and alleviate coughing may be recommended.

Oxygen Therapy: In severe cases, supplemental oxygen may be provided to ensure adequate oxygen levels in the blood.

Prevention

Vaccination: Vaccines are available to prevent some of the common causes of pneumonia, such as the pneumococcal vaccine and the influenza vaccine.

Good Hygiene Practices: Regular handwashing, avoiding close contact with sick individuals, and practicing good respiratory hygiene can help prevent the spread of infections.

Healthy Lifestyle: Maintaining overall health, including a balanced diet, regular exercise, and adequate sleep, can contribute to a strong immune system.

Complications

Complications of pneumonia can include respiratory failure, sepsis, pleural effusion (fluid accumulation around the lungs), and lung abscesses. The risk of complications is higher in older adults, young children, and individuals with weakened immune systems.

Prompt diagnosis and appropriate treatment are crucial for a positive outcome in pneumonia. Individuals with severe symptoms, such as difficulty breathing, persistent chest pain, or high fever, should seek medical attention promptly. Most cases of pneumonia can be effectively treated with appropriate medical care, but severe cases may require hospitalization.

Cystic Fibrosis

Cystic fibrosis (CF) is a genetic disorder that primarily affects the respiratory and digestive systems. It is caused by mutations in the CFTR gene, which leads to the production of thick and sticky mucus. This mucus can block the airways and ducts, leading to a range of respiratory and digestive problems. Cystic fibrosis is a chronic condition, and its severity can vary widely among individuals.

Key Features of Cystic Fibrosis:
Respiratory System Involvement:

•Thick Mucus: The abnormally thick and sticky mucus clogs the airways, making it difficult to breathe and leading to chronic lung infections.
•Chronic Bronchitis: Recurrent inflammation of the airways and persistent coughing with mucus production.
Digestive System Involvement:

•Pancreatic Insufficiency: Thickened mucus can block the pancreatic ducts, leading to a lack of digestive enzymes and difficulties in digesting and absorbing nutrients.

•Malabsorption: Inadequate nutrient absorption can result in poor weight gain, malnutrition, and vitamin deficiencies.

Other Manifestations

•Sweat Gland Dysfunction: Individuals with CF have saltier sweat than normal, which can be used as a diagnostic tool.

•Sinus and Nasal Issues: Chronic sinusitis and nasal polyps are common in people with CF.

Genetic Basis:

•Autosomal Recessive Inheritance: Cystic fibrosis is inherited in an autosomal recessive manner, meaning that an individual must inherit a mutated CFTR gene from both parents to develop the condition.

•CFTR Gene Mutations: There are many different mutations in the CFTR gene, with some being more common than others. The type of mutation can influence the severity of symptoms and the progression of the disease.Diagnosis:

•Newborn Screening: Many countries include cystic fibrosis in their newborn screening programs, allowing for early detection and intervention.

•Sweat Test: The gold standard for diagnosing CF is the sweat test, which measures the concentration of salt in sweat. People with CF have elevated levels of salt.

•Genetic Testing: Identification of CFTR gene mutations through genetic testing can confirm the diagnosis.

Treatment

•Airway Clearance Techniques: Physical therapy techniques and devices to help clear mucus from the airways.

•Bronchodilators: Medications to help relax the muscles around the airways.

•Antibiotics: Prescribed to treat and prevent respiratory infections.

•Pancreatic Enzyme Replacement: Enzyme supplements to aid digestion and nutrient absorption.

•Nutritional Support: Specialized diets, nutritional supplements, and, in severe cases, tube feeding may be necessary.

•Lung Transplant: In advanced cases, a lung transplant may be considered.

Prognosis

Advances in medical care and treatments have significantly improved the life expectancy and quality of life for individuals with cystic fibrosis. However, it remains a chronic and progressive condition. The severity of symptoms can vary, and ongoing medical care, including medications, physiotherapy, and nutritional support, is essential to manage the disease and improve outcomes. Early diagnosis and intervention play a crucial role in providing the best possible care for individuals with cystic fibrosis.

Obstructive Sleep Apnea (OSA)

Obstructive Sleep Apnea (OSA) is a sleep disorder characterized by repeated episodes of partial or complete blockage of the upper airway during sleep. These episodes, known as apneas, lead to disruptions in breathing and can result in a range of symptoms and potential health consequences. OSA is one of the most common sleep disorders.

Key Features of Obstructive Sleep Apnea:
•Airway Obstruction:

During sleep, the muscles in the throat and tongue relax. In individuals with OSA, these muscles relax excessively, causing a narrowing or complete closure of the upper airway.
•Breathing Pauses (Apneas):

The airway obstruction leads to temporary pauses in breathing, typically lasting for 10 seconds or longer. These pauses can occur multiple times per hour throughout the night.
•Micro-Arousals:

Each breathing pause is often accompanied by a partial awakening or arousal from deep sleep as the brain signals the body to resume breathing.

Risk Factors

•Obesity: Excess weight, especially around the neck, increases the risk of airway obstruction.

•Neck Circumference: Individuals with a thicker neck circumference may be more prone to airway narrowing.

•Gender: Men are more commonly affected than women, though the risk in women increases if they are overweight.

•Age: OSA is more prevalent in older adults.

•Family History: There may be a genetic predisposition to OSA.

•Medical Conditions: Conditions such as hypertension, diabetes, and certain neurological disorders can increase the risk.

Symptoms

•Loud Snoring: Often a prominent symptom, though not everyone who snores has OSA.

•Pauses in Breathing: Reported by a bed partner or observed during sleep.

•Excessive Daytime Sleepiness: Due to disrupted sleep and frequent awakenings.

•Morning Headaches: Caused by the impact of interrupted breathing on oxygen levels.

•Difficulty Concentrating: Cognitive impairment and memory issues can occur.

•Irritability and Mood Changes: Disrupted sleep can affect mood and overall well-being.

Diagnosis

•Sleep Study (Polysomnography): The most common diagnostic test involves monitoring various physiological parameters during a night's sleep. This can be done either in a sleep center or at home with portable devices.

•Home Sleep Apnea Test (HSAT): A simplified version of polysomnography that can be used in certain cases to diagnose OSA.

Treatment

•Continuous Positive Airway Pressure (CPAP): The most common and effective treatment. A CPAP machine delivers a constant stream of air through a mask to keep the airway open.

•Bi-level Positive Airway Pressure (BiPAP): Similar to CPAP but provides different pressures for inhalation and exhalation, which can be more comfortable for some individuals.

•Positive Airway Pressure (PAP) Therapy: Other devices, such as automatic positive airway pressure (APAP) machines, may be used based on individual needs.

•Oral Appliances: Dental devices that reposition the lower jaw and tongue to keep the airway open.

•Lifestyle Changes: Weight loss, positional therapy, and avoiding alcohol and sedatives before bedtime.

•Surgery: In some cases, surgical procedures such as uvulopalatopharyngoplasty (UPPP) or genioglossus advancement (GA) may be considered.

Complications

Untreated OSA can lead to various health issues, including cardiovascular problems (hypertension, heart disease), diabetes, cognitive impairment, and an increased risk of accidents due to daytime sleepiness.

♦Early diagnosis and appropriate treatment are crucial for managing OSA and preventing its associated complications. Individuals experiencing symptoms of OSA should seek evaluation and diagnosis from a healthcare professional, usually a sleep specialist.

Lung Cancer

Lung cancer is a type of cancer that begins in the lungs, usually in the cells lining the air passages. It is one of the most common types of cancer globally and a leading cause of cancer-related deaths. There are two main types of lung cancer: **non-small cell lung cancer (NSCLC) and small cell lung cancer (SCLC).** NSCLC is more common, accounting for about 85% of all cases, while SCLC tends to be more aggressive.

Causes and Risk Factors

•Smoking: Cigarette smoking is the leading cause of lung cancer. The risk is directly related to the duration of smoking and the number of cigarettes smoked.

•Secondhand Smoke: Non-smokers exposed to secondhand smoke are also at an increased risk of developing lung cancer.

•Occupational Exposures: Certain occupations, such as asbestos workers, miners, and those exposed to radon or certain chemicals, may have an elevated risk.

•Family History: A family history of lung cancer may increase the risk, suggesting a potential genetic component.

•Previous Lung Diseases: Individuals with a history of certain lung diseases, such as chronic obstructive pulmonary disease (COPD), are at an increased risk.

Types of Lung Cancer

♦Non-Small Cell Lung Cancer (NSCLC):

•Adenocarcinoma: Most common type, often found in the outer regions of the lungs. It is more common in non-smokers and women.
Squamous Cell Carcinoma: Usually found in the central airways. Linked to a history of smoking.
•Large Cell Carcinoma: Can occur in any part of the lung. Tends to grow and spread quickly.
♦Small Cell Lung Cancer (SCLC):

•Extensive Stage: Often diagnosed after it has already spread beyond the lungs.
Limited Stage: Confined to one lung and possibly nearby lymph nodes.

Symptoms

•Persistent Cough: A cough that doesn't go away or worsens over time.

•Shortness of Breath: Difficulty breathing or wheezing.

•Chest Pain: Pain in the chest, shoulders, or back unrelated to coughing.

•Unexplained Weight Loss: Significant and unintentional weight loss.

•Hoarseness: Changes in the voice or persistent hoarseness.

•Recurrent Infections: Frequent respiratory infections, such as bronchitis or pneumonia.

Diagnosis

Imaging Studies:

•Chest X-ray: Often the initial test to detect abnormalities.
•CT Scan: Provides detailed images to assess the size and location of tumors.
•Biopsy:

Bronchoscopy: A thin, flexible tube with a camera is used to view the airways and collect tissue samples.
•Needle Biopsy: A needle is used to extract a tissue sample from the lung.
•Staging:

Determines the extent of cancer spread, influencing treatment decisions.

Treatment

•Surgery: Removal of the tumor and surrounding tissue may be an option for early-stage lung cancer.

•Radiation Therapy: Uses high-energy rays to target and kill cancer cells.

•Chemotherapy: Medications to kill cancer cells or slow their growth.

•Targeted Therapy: Targets specific molecules involved in cancer growth.

•Immunotherapy: Boosts the body's immune system to fight cancer cells.

Prognosis

The prognosis for lung cancer depends on various factors, including the stage at diagnosis, the type of cancer, the person's overall health, and the effectiveness of treatment. Early detection and intervention generally improve outcomes. However, lung cancer is often diagnosed at an advanced stage, which can limit treatment options and affect survival rates. Quitting smoking and avoiding exposure to tobacco smoke and other environmental risk factors can significantly reduce the risk of developing lung cancer.

Chapter 3
Neurological conditions

Neurological conditions refer to disorders that affect the nervous system, which includes the brain, spinal cord, and nerves throughout the body. The nervous system is responsible for coordinating and controlling various bodily functions, and when it malfunctions, it can lead to a wide range of symptoms and health issues. Neurological conditions can be broadly categorized into several types, including:

Degenerative Disorders: These conditions involve the gradual loss or deterioration of nerve cells. Examples include Alzheimer's disease, Parkinson's disease, and amyotrophic lateral sclerosis (ALS).

Inflammatory Disorders: Conditions that involve inflammation of the nervous system. Multiple sclerosis (MS) is an example where the immune system mistakenly attacks the protective covering of nerve fibers.

Vascular Disorders: Conditions related to problems with blood flow to the brain or spinal cord. Stroke is a common vascular disorder that can result in neurological deficits.

Traumatic Injuries: Injuries to the nervous system due to trauma, such as traumatic brain injury (TBI) or spinal cord injury. These injuries can have a wide range of effects depending on the location and severity of the trauma.

Epilepsy: Characterized by recurrent seizures due to abnormal electrical activity in the brain.The symptoms of neurological conditions can vary widely, depending on the specific disorder and the affected area of the nervous system. Common symptoms include changes in sensation, movement, cognition, and behavior.

Diagnosis often involves a combination of medical history, physical examination, imaging studies (like MRI or CT scans), and sometimes specialized tests like electroencephalography (EEG) or nerve conduction studies.

Treatment for neurological conditions depends on the specific disorder and may include medications, physical therapy, surgery, and supportive care.

Additionally, ongoing research aims to discover new treatments and improve our understanding of these complex conditions.

Degenerative Disorders

Degenerative disorders are a category of medical conditions characterized by the gradual deterioration or loss of the structure and function of tissues or organs over time. These disorders often progress slowly and may be associated with aging, although they can also have genetic, environmental, or unknown causes. The degeneration typically involves a breakdown of cells, tissues, or organs, leading to a decline in their normal functioning. One prominent area where degenerative disorders occur is in the nervous system. Here are some key points about degenerative disorders:

Neurodegenerative Disorders

Examples: Alzheimer's disease, Parkinson's disease, Huntington's disease, and amyotrophic lateral sclerosis (ALS).

Characteristics: These disorders involve the progressive degeneration of nerve cells, leading to a decline in cognitive function (in the case of Alzheimer's), movement control (in the case of Parkinson's and Huntington's), or motor function (in the case of ALS).

Musculoskeletal Degeneration

Examples: Osteoarthritis, degenerative disc disease.
Characteristics: Involves the gradual breakdown of joint cartilage (osteoarthritis) or intervertebral discs in the spine (degenerative disc disease), leading to pain, stiffness, and reduced mobility.

Cardiovascular Degeneration:

Example: Atherosclerosis.
Characteristics: Atherosclerosis is a condition in which fatty deposits build up on the walls of arteries over time, leading to a narrowing and hardening of the arteries. This can restrict blood flow and contribute to cardiovascular diseases.

Retinal Degeneration

Example: Age-related macular degeneration.
Characteristics: This disorder affects the retina, leading to a gradual loss of central vision, often associated with aging.

Genetic Degenerative Disorders

Example: Cystic fibrosis.

Characteristics: Some degenerative disorders have a genetic basis, where mutations in specific genes lead to the progressive degeneration of certain tissues or organs. In the case of cystic fibrosis, it affects the respiratory and digestive systems.

Hormonal Degeneration:

Example: Menopause.

Characteristics: While not a disorder in the traditional sense, menopause is a natural process involving the gradual decline in reproductive hormones in women, leading to various physiological changes.

Cellular Degeneration:

Example: Cellular senescence.

Characteristics: Cellular senescence refers to the process by which cells lose their ability to divide and function over time. It is associated with aging and contributes to the overall aging process.

Management and treatment of degenerative disorders often focus on alleviating symptoms, slowing down the progression of the degeneration, and improving the individual's quality of life. Depending on the specific disorder, interventions may include medications, physical therapy, lifestyle modifications, and in some cases, surgical procedures. Research continues to explore ways to better understand these disorders and develop more effective treatments.

Inflammatory Disorders

Inflammatory disorders are conditions characterized by an abnormal and excessive immune response, leading to inflammation in various tissues and organs of the body. Inflammation is a natural and protective response that the body employs to defend itself against harmful stimuli, such as pathogens, damaged cells, or irritants. However, in inflammatory disorders, this immune response becomes dysregulated, causing inflammation to persist and even target the body's own tissues. Chronic inflammation can contribute to tissue damage and a range of symptoms. Here are some key points about inflammatory disorders:

Autoimmune Inflammatory Disorders:

Examples: Rheumatoid arthritis, systemic lupus erythematosus (SLE), inflammatory bowel diseases (Crohn's disease and ulcerative colitis).

Characteristics: In autoimmune disorders, the immune system mistakenly recognizes the body's own tissues as foreign and mounts an inflammatory response against them. This can lead to joint inflammation (as in rheumatoid arthritis), skin rashes (as in lupus), or inflammation in the gastrointestinal tract (as in inflammatory bowel diseases).

Allergic Inflammatory Disorders:

Examples: Allergic rhinitis, asthma, atopic dermatitis.

Characteristics: Allergic reactions involve an immune response to harmless substances (allergens) such as pollen, dust, or certain foods. The immune system releases inflammatory chemicals, leading to symptoms like sneezing, itching, difficulty breathing, or skin rashes.

Chronic Inflammatory Diseases:

Examples: Chronic obstructive pulmonary disease (COPD), atherosclerosis.

Characteristics: Conditions like COPD and atherosclerosis involve persistent inflammation that contributes to tissue damage over time. In COPD, inflammation in the airways can lead to breathing difficulties, while atherosclerosis involves inflammation in the arteries, contributing to the development of plaques that can narrow and block blood vessels.

Inflammatory Skin Disorders

Examples: Psoriasis, eczema (dermatitis).

Characteristics: Skin disorders characterized by inflammation, redness, and itching. In psoriasis, there is an overactive immune response that leads to the rapid turnover of skin cells, resulting in thick, scaly patches. Eczema involves inflammation of the skin, causing itching and a rash.

Neuroinflammatory Disorders

Examples: Multiple sclerosis, encephalitis.

Characteristics: Inflammation in the nervous system can lead to conditions like multiple sclerosis, where the protective covering of nerve fibers is damaged, or encephalitis, which involves inflammation of the brain.

Infectious Inflammatory Disorders

Examples: Meningitis, sepsis.

Characteristics: Infections can trigger a robust inflammatory response. In meningitis, the protective membranes covering the brain and spinal cord become inflamed. Sepsis is a systemic inflammatory response to severe infection that can lead to organ dysfunction.

Treatment of inflammatory disorders often involves managing the immune response to reduce inflammation and alleviate symptoms. Medications such as nonsteroidal anti-inflammatory drugs (NSAIDs), corticosteroids, disease-modifying antirheumatic drugs (DMARDs), and biologics may be prescribed. Lifestyle modifications, including diet and exercise, can also play a role in managing inflammation. The specific approach depends on the type and severity of the inflammatory disorders.

Vascular disorders

Vascular disorders refer to a group of conditions that affect the blood vessels, including arteries, veins, and capillaries. These disorders can disrupt the normal flow of blood and may lead to various complications depending on the location and severity of the vascular issues.

types of vascular disorders:

Atherosclerosis:

Characteristics: Atherosclerosis is a common vascular disorder characterized by the accumulation of fatty deposits, cholesterol, and other substances on the inner walls of arteries. This can lead to the formation of plaques that narrow and harden the arteries, restricting blood flow. Atherosclerosis is a major contributor to cardiovascular diseases, such as coronary artery disease and peripheral arterial disease.

Peripheral Arterial Disease (PAD):

Characteristics: PAD is a type of atherosclerosis that affects the arteries supplying blood to the extremities, usually the legs. Reduced blood flow to the legs can cause pain, cramping, and difficulties with walking. In severe cases, PAD can lead to tissue damage and non-healing ulcers.

Aneurysm:

Characteristics: An aneurysm is a bulge or ballooning in the wall of a blood vessel. Aneurysms can occur in various arteries, but they are particularly concerning when they affect the aorta (the largest artery in the body) or brain. If an aneurysm ruptures, it can lead to life-threatening bleeding.

Hypertension (High Blood Pressure):

Characteristics: Chronic high blood pressure can damage the walls of arteries, making them more prone to atherosclerosis and increasing the risk of cardiovascular events such as heart attack and stroke. Hypertension is a common vascular disorder that often coexists with other cardiovascular conditions.

Venous Thrombosis:

Characteristics: This includes deep vein thrombosis (DVT) and superficial vein thrombosis. DVT occurs when a blood clot forms in a deep vein, often in the legs. If a clot breaks loose and travels to the lungs, it can cause a pulmonary embolism. Superficial vein thrombosis involves blood clot formation in veins closer to the skin's surface.

Varicose Veins:

Characteristics: Varicose veins are enlarged, twisted veins that often occur in the legs. They result from weakened valves in the veins, which can lead to pooling of blood and increased pressure. Varicose veins are usually a cosmetic concern but can cause discomfort.

Raynaud's Disease:

Characteristics: Raynaud's disease is characterized by episodes of reduced blood flow to certain parts of the body, usually the fingers and toes, in response to cold or stress. This can lead to color changes in the affected areas and may cause pain or numbness.

Vasculitis:

Characteristics: Vasculitis is an inflammation of the blood vessels. It can affect vessels of any size, and symptoms vary depending on the type and location of the affected vessels. Vasculitis can be a primary condition or secondary to other autoimmune diseases.

Treatment for vascular disorders depends on the specific condition and its severity. Interventions may include lifestyle modifications (such as diet and exercise), medications to manage blood pressure or prevent clot formation, and, in some cases, surgical procedures to repair or bypass affected vessels. Early diagnosis and management are crucial to prevent complications and improve outcomes for individuals with vascular disorders.

Traumatic Injuries

Traumatic injuries refer to physical injuries or damage to the body that result from an external force or impact. These injuries can occur suddenly and are often the consequence of accidents, falls, collisions, or other events that expose the body to mechanical forces beyond its tolerance. Traumatic injuries can affect various parts of the body, and their severity can range from minor cuts and bruises to life-threatening conditions.

Common types of traumatic injuries:

Soft Tissue Injuries:

Examples: Contusions (bruises), abrasions (scrapes), lacerations (cuts), and sprains.
Characteristics: Soft tissue injuries involve damage to the skin, muscles, ligaments, and tendons. Contusions and abrasions are often superficial, while lacerations can penetrate deeper tissues. Sprains involve the stretching or tearing of ligaments.

Fractures (Bone Injuries):

Examples: Broken bones.
Characteristics: Fractures occur when the force applied to a bone is stronger than the bone itself can withstand. Fractures can be simple (a clean break) or compound (the bone pierces the skin), and they may require immobilization, casting, or surgical intervention for proper healing.

Head Injuries:

Examples: Concussions, contusions, skull fractures.
Characteristics: Head injuries can result from falls, motor vehicle accidents, or blunt force trauma to the head. Concussions are a type of head injury

involving temporary impairment of brain function, while contusions and fractures involve damage to the skull and brain tissues.

Spinal Cord Injuries:

Characteristics: Injuries to the spinal cord can result in the loss of sensation, muscle function, or both, below the level of the injury. These injuries can lead to paralysis or significant motor and sensory impairments.

Burn Injuries:

Characteristics: Burns can result from exposure to heat, chemicals, electricity, or radiation. The severity of burns is classified into degrees (first, second, and third), with third-degree burns involving the full thickness of the skin and potentially underlying tissues.

Traumatic Amputations:

Characteristics: Traumatic amputations involve the partial or complete loss of a body part due to injury. These injuries often require immediate medical attention and may involve surgical intervention to control bleeding and repair damaged tissues.

Internal Injuries:

Examples: Internal bleeding, organ damage.

Characteristics: Trauma can cause damage to internal organs, leading to bleeding or other complications. Internal injuries may not be immediately visible, and their severity may require diagnostic imaging, such as CT scans, to assess the extent of damage.

Crush Injuries:

Characteristics: Crush injuries occur when a body part is subjected to a high amount of force or pressure, often resulting in damage to muscles, nerves, and blood vessels. These injuries can be associated with events like car accidents or industrial accidents.

Facial Injuries:

Examples: Fractures of the facial bones, dental injuries.

Characteristics: Trauma to the face can result in fractures of the bones in the facial skeleton, such as the nose or jaw. Injuries to the teeth and soft tissues of the face are also common.

Thoracic and Abdominal Injuries:

Characteristics: Trauma to the chest or abdomen can lead to injuries to the organs in these regions, such as the lungs, heart, liver, or spleen. These injuries may be caused by blunt force trauma or penetrating injuries.

♦Immediate and appropriate medical care is crucial for individuals with traumatic injuries. Treatment may involve first aid, immobilization, surgery, medications, rehabilitation, and long-term medical management, depending on the type and severity of the injury. Early intervention can significantly impact the outcome and recovery of individuals with traumatic injuries.

Epilepsy

Epilepsy is a neurological disorder characterized by recurrent, unprovoked seizures. A seizure is a sudden, temporary disturbance in the brain's electrical activity, leading to various symptoms and behaviors. Seizures can vary widely in their presentation and impact on individuals, and they may involve alterations in consciousness, movements, sensations, or a combination of these.

Types

•**Seizure Types:**

Generalized Seizures: Involve widespread electrical activity in the brain and affect both hemispheres.

Tonic-Clonic (Grand Mal) Seizures: Involves loss of consciousness, stiffening of muscles (tonic phase), followed by rhythmic jerking movements (clonic phase).

Absence Seizures: Brief loss of consciousness with a blank stare; often seen in children.

Myoclonic Seizures: Sudden, brief jerking or twitching of muscles.

Focal (Partial) Seizures: Originate in a specific area of the brain and may or may not spread to involve the entire brain.

Simple Partial Seizures: Cause localized symptoms without loss of consciousness.

Complex Partial Seizures: Involve altered consciousness and complex, purposeless movements.

Secondary Generalized Seizures: Begin as focal seizures and evolve into generalized seizures.

Causes and Triggers

Idiopathic: The cause is unknown, and it is believed to have a genetic basis.

Symptomatic or Secondary: Caused by an identifiable underlying condition, such as brain injury, infection, stroke, or tumors.

Triggers: Seizures can be triggered by factors like stress, lack of sleep, flashing lights (photosensitivity), or specific medications.
Diagnosis:

Diagnosis is typically based on a thorough medical history, neurological examination, and diagnostic tests, including electroencephalogram (EEG), which records the brain's electrical activity during seizures.

Treatment

Medications: Antiepileptic drugs (AEDs) are the most common treatment and are tailored to the specific type of seizures. Finding the right medication and dosage may require adjustments.
Lifestyle Modifications: Ensuring sufficient sleep, managing stress, and avoiding seizure triggers can help reduce the frequency of seizures.
Surgery: In some cases, surgery may be considered to remove or disconnect the area of the brain causing seizures.
Vagus Nerve Stimulation (VNS): A device implanted under the skin stimulates the vagus nerve to help prevent seizures.
Ketogenic Diet: A high-fat, low-carbohydrate diet may be recommended for some individuals, especially children.

Impact on Daily Life

Epilepsy can impact various aspects of daily life, including education, employment, and social interactions. Stigma associated with epilepsy can contribute to challenges in personal and social well-being.

Prognosis

Many individuals with epilepsy can effectively manage their condition with medications and lifestyle adjustments. Some may outgrow epilepsy, especially if the onset occurs in childhood. In some cases, epilepsy may be more challenging to control, and seizures may persist despite treatment.

Safety Considerations

Safety is a significant concern for individuals with epilepsy. Precautions may include avoiding activities with a high risk of injury during seizures, such as swimming alone or working at heights.

Public Awareness and Advocacy:

Public awareness about epilepsy is crucial to dispel myths and reduce stigma. Advocacy efforts aim to improve understanding, access to care, and support for individuals with epilepsy.

♦It's important for individuals with epilepsy to work closely with healthcare professionals to manage their condition effectively. Regular medical follow-ups, adherence to prescribed medications, and open communication about symptoms and concerns contribute to better seizure control and overall well-being.

Chapter 4

Psychiatric conditions

Psychiatric conditions, also known as mental health disorders or illnesses, are a broad range of conditions that affect a person's thinking, feeling, behavior, or mood. These conditions can significantly impact a person's ability to function in daily life, maintain relationships, and handle stress. Psychiatric conditions can be caused by a variety of factors, including biological, psychological, and environmental influences.

Common psychiatric conditions:

Depressive Disorders: Conditions characterized by persistent feelings of sadness, hopelessness, and a lack of interest or pleasure in activities. Major depressive disorder, bipolar disorder, and persistent depressive disorder are examples.

Anxiety Disorders: Conditions involving excessive worry, fear, or nervousness. Examples include generalized anxiety disorder, panic disorder, social anxiety disorder, and specific phobias.

Schizophrenia Spectrum and Other Psychotic Disorders: These conditions involve disruptions in thinking, perception, and behavior. Individuals may experience hallucinations, delusions, and impaired cognitive function.

Obsessive-Compulsive and Related Disorders: Conditions characterized by persistent, intrusive thoughts (obsessions) and repetitive behaviors or mental acts (compulsions) performed to reduce anxiety.

Trauma- and Stressor-Related Disorders: Conditions related to exposure to traumatic or stressful events. Post-traumatic stress disorder (PTSD) is a common example.

Substance-Related and Addictive Disorders: Conditions related to the use of substances (such as drugs or alcohol) that lead to significant impairment or distress.

Understanding that psychiatric disorders are intricate, their distinctions aren't consistently straightforward. Furthermore, individuals might grapple with multiple conditions simultaneously, a state referred to as comorbidity. Effective treatments typically entail a blend of therapy, medication, and lifestyle adjustments customized to meet individual needs. It's vital to seek guidance from mental health experts—be it psychiatrists, psychologists, or counselors—for precise diagnosis and successful treatment.

Depressive Disorders

Depressive disorders are a category of mental health conditions characterized by persistent feelings of sadness, hopelessness, and a lack of interest or pleasure in activities. These conditions significantly impact a person's daily life, relationships, work, and overall functioning. Depressive disorders are common, affecting millions of people worldwide, and they can vary in severity and duration.

Common types of depressive disorders:

Major Depressive Disorder (MDD): Also known as clinical depression, MDD involves a persistent and intense low mood that lasts for at least two weeks. Symptoms include a diminished interest in activities, changes in appetite or weight, sleep disturbances, fatigue, feelings of worthlessness or guilt, difficulty concentrating, and thoughts of death or suicide.

Persistent Depressive Disorder (Dysthymia): Dysthymia is characterized by a chronic, long-term form of depression. While the symptoms are not as severe as those in major depressive disorder, they persist for at least two years in adults (one year in children and adolescents).

Bipolar Disorder: Bipolar disorder, previously known as manic-depressive illness, involves alternating periods of depressive episodes and manic or hypomanic episodes. During manic episodes, individuals may experience elevated mood, increased energy, impulsivity, and a reduced need for sleep.

Seasonal Affective Disorder (SAD): This type of depression occurs at a specific time of the year, usually during the fall and winter months when there is less natural sunlight. Symptoms include low energy, irritability, difficulty concentrating, changes in sleep and appetite, and a craving for carbohydrates.

Postpartum Depression: Experienced by some women after giving birth, postpartum depression involves intense feelings of sadness, anxiety, and exhaustion that can interfere with the ability to care for oneself and the newborn.

Premenstrual Dysphoric Disorder (PMDD): This is a severe form of premenstrual syndrome (PMS) that includes significant mood disturbances, such as depression, irritability, and tension, in the weeks leading up to menstruation.

The exact causes of depressive disorders are complex and often involve a combination of genetic, biological, environmental, and psychological factors. Imbalances in neurotransmitters, such as serotonin and norepinephrine, are commonly implicated in depressive disorders.

Treatment for depressive disorders typically involves a combination of approaches:

•Psychotherapy: Cognitive-behavioral therapy (CBT), interpersonal therapy (IPT), and other therapeutic approaches can help individuals explore and manage their thoughts, feelings, and behaviors.

•Medication: Antidepressant medications, such as selective serotonin reuptake inhibitors (SSRIs) or serotonin-norepinephrine reuptake inhibitors (SNRIs), may be prescribed to help regulate neurotransmitter levels.

•Lifestyle Changes: Regular exercise, a healthy diet, sufficient sleep, and stress management can contribute to improved mood and overall well-being.

•Support Groups: Connecting with others who are experiencing similar challenges can provide valuable support and understanding.

It's important for individuals experiencing symptoms of depression to seek professional help. A mental health professional can provide an accurate diagnosis and work with the individual to develop a personalized treatment plan. In severe cases, hospitalization may be necessary to ensure the safety of the individual. If you or someone you know is struggling with depression, it's crucial to reach out to a healthcare provider or mental health professional for assistance.

Anxiety Disorders

Anxiety disorders are a group of mental health conditions characterized by excessive and persistent worry, fear, or apprehension. These feelings can be overwhelming and interfere with daily life, affecting an individual's thoughts, emotions, and behaviors. Anxiety disorders are among the most common mental health disorders, and they can manifest in various forms.

Some common types of anxiety disorders:

Generalized Anxiety Disorder (GAD): GAD involves chronic and excessive worry about a wide range of events or activities. Individuals with GAD often find it challenging to control their worry, and they may experience physical symptoms such as restlessness, muscle tension, fatigue, irritability, and sleep disturbances.

Panic Disorder: Panic disorder is characterized by recurring and unexpected panic attacks, which are sudden episodes of intense fear accompanied by physical symptoms such as heart palpitations, sweating, trembling, shortness of breath, and a sense of impending doom. Individuals with panic disorder often develop a fear of future panic attacks, leading to avoidance behaviors.

Social Anxiety Disorder (Social Phobia): Social anxiety disorder involves an intense fear of social situations, where individuals may feel judged, embarrassed, or humiliated. This fear can lead to avoidance of social interactions, negatively impacting personal and professional relationships.

Specific Phobias: These are intense, irrational fears of specific objects or situations. Common phobias include fear of heights (acrophobia), fear of spiders (arachnophobia), and fear of flying (aviophobia).

Individuals with specific phobias may go to great lengths to avoid the feared stimulus.

Obsessive-Compulsive Disorder (OCD): OCD is characterized by intrusive, unwanted thoughts (obsessions) and repetitive behaviors or mental rituals (compulsions) performed in an attempt to reduce anxiety. Common obsessions include fears of contamination, harm coming to oneself or others, or a need for symmetry.

Post-Traumatic Stress Disorder (PTSD): PTSD can develop following exposure to a traumatic event, such as combat, sexual assault, or a natural disaster. Symptoms include intrusive memories, flashbacks, nightmares, hypervigilance, and avoidance of reminders of the trauma.

Agoraphobia: Agoraphobia involves an intense fear of being in situations or places where escape might be difficult or embarrassing, leading to avoidance of these situations. It can often co-occur with panic disorder.

Anxiety disorders can have various causes, including a combination of genetic, biological, environmental, and psychological factors. Traumatic experiences, chronic stress, and a family history of anxiety disorders can contribute to their development.

Treatments

Psychotherapy: Cognitive-behavioral therapy (CBT) is particularly effective in addressing distorted thought patterns and maladaptive behaviors associated with anxiety disorders.

Medication: Antidepressants, benzodiazepines, and other medications may be prescribed to help alleviate symptoms, particularly in cases of severe anxiety.

Lifestyle Changes: Regular exercise, adequate sleep, and stress management techniques can contribute to overall well-being and help manage anxiety.

Support Groups: Connecting with others who experience similar challenges can provide valuable support and understanding.

♦It's important for individuals experiencing symptoms of anxiety to seek professional help. A mental health professional can provide an accurate diagnosis and work with the individual to develop a personalized treatment plan.

Obsessive-Compulsive and Related Disorders

Obsessive-Compulsive and Related Disorders are a category of mental health conditions characterized by the presence of obsessive thoughts, compulsive behaviors, or a combination of both. These disorders are outlined in the Diagnostic and Statistical Manual of Mental Disorders, Fifth Edition (DSM-5), which is a widely used classification system for mental health disorders.

Some key Obsessive-Compulsive and Related Disorders:

Obsessive-Compulsive Disorder (OCD): OCD is characterized by the presence of obsessions and compulsions. Obsessions are intrusive and unwanted thoughts, images, or urges that cause significant anxiety or distress. Compulsions are repetitive behaviors or mental acts performed to alleviate the distress associated with the obsessions. Common themes include contamination fears, fears of harming oneself or others, and a need for symmetry or order.

Body Dysmorphic Disorder (BDD): Individuals with BDD are preoccupied with perceived flaws or defects in their physical appearance, which are often minor or imagined. This preoccupation leads to significant distress and impairment in daily functioning. Compulsive behaviors may include excessive grooming, seeking reassurance, or comparing oneself to others.

Hoarding Disorder: Hoarding disorder is characterized by persistent difficulty parting with possessions, regardless of their actual value. Individuals with hoarding disorder accumulate a large number of items, leading to clutter that significantly impairs living spaces. This behavior can result in distress and functional impairment.

Trichotillomania (Hair-Pulling Disorder): Trichotillomania involves recurrent pulling out of one's hair, leading to noticeable hair loss. Individuals with this disorder may experience tension before pulling and a sense of relief or gratification afterward. Trichotillomania can result in significant distress and impairment in social, occupational, or other areas of functioning.

Excoriation (Skin-Picking) Disorder: Also known as dermatillomania, this disorder involves recurrent picking at one's skin, leading to skin lesions.

Similar to trichotillomania, individuals may feel tension before picking and relief afterward. The behavior can lead to physical harm and impairment in daily life.

Obsessive-Compulsive and Related Disorder Due to Another Medical Condition: This category includes conditions where obsessive-compulsive or related symptoms are a direct result of a medical condition, such as a neurological disorder or infection.

These disorders share common features of intrusive and distressing thoughts and repetitive behaviors that individuals feel compelled to perform. The severity of symptoms can vary, and the impact on daily functioning may range from mild to severe.

Treatment for Obsessive-Compulsive and Related Disorders often involves a combination of **psychotherapy**, **medication**, and **support**. Cognitive-behavioral therapy (CBT), particularly exposure and response prevention (ERP), is a widely used and effective therapeutic approach for managing these disorders. Medications, such as selective serotonin reuptake inhibitors (SSRIs), may also be prescribed to alleviate symptoms.

♦It's important for individuals experiencing symptoms of these disorders to seek professional help. A mental health professional can provide an accurate diagnosis and work with the individual to develop a personalized treatment plan.

Substance-Related and Addictive Disorders

Substance-Related and Addictive Disorders refer to a group of mental health conditions characterized by problematic patterns of substance use, leading to significant impairment or distress. These disorders encompass a range of substances, including alcohol, prescription medications, and illicit drugs. They are outlined in the Diagnostic and Statistical Manual of Mental Disorders, Fifth Edition (DSM-5), which is a widely used classification system for mental health disorders.

Key Substance-Related and Addictive Disorders:

Substance Use Disorder (SUD): This is a broad category that includes disorders related to the use of substances, including alcohol, cannabis, stimulants, opioids, and others. Substance Use Disorder is characterized by a cluster of symptoms that indicate impaired control over substance use, social impairment, risky use, and pharmacological criteria (tolerance and withdrawal).

Alcohol Use Disorder (AUD): This specific disorder focuses on problematic alcohol use. Individuals with AUD may exhibit behaviors such as drinking in larger amounts or for a longer period than intended, unsuccessful attempts to cut down or control drinking, and continued use despite adverse consequences.

Opioid Use Disorder: This disorder pertains to the problematic use of opioids, including prescription painkillers and illicit substances like heroin. Symptoms include a strong desire to use opioids, unsuccessful attempts to control use, and continued use despite negative consequences.

Stimulant Use Disorder: This disorder involves the problematic use of stimulant drugs such as cocaine or methamphetamine. Symptoms may include increased tolerance, cravings, and spending a significant amount of time obtaining or using the substance.

Cannabis Use Disorder: This disorder is related to problematic cannabis use, characterized by symptoms such as unsuccessful efforts to cut down use, continued use despite negative consequences, and neglect of important activities.

Tobacco Use Disorder: While not a substance use disorder in the DSM-5, the addictive nature of nicotine is recognized, and tobacco use disorders are commonly discussed. Symptoms include a persistent desire to quit or cut down on tobacco use but being unable to do so.

Gambling Disorder: Although not directly related to substance use, Gambling Disorder is categorized under the broader umbrella of Addictive Disorders. It involves persistent and problematic gambling behavior that leads to significant impairment or distress.

Treatment for Substance-Related and Addictive Disorders often involves a combination of ***behavioral therapies, counseling, support groups***, and, in some cases, ***medication***. The goals of treatment include reducing or eliminating substance use, addressing underlying issues contributing to the disorder, and helping individuals build healthier coping mechanisms.

Recovery from substance-related disorders is often a complex and ongoing process, and relapse prevention is a crucial component of treatment. Seeking help from mental health professionals, addiction specialists, or support groups can significantly improve the chances of successful recovery.

Trauma- and Stressor-Related Disorders

Trauma- and Stressor-Related Disorders encompass a group of mental health conditions that develop following exposure to traumatic or highly stressful events. These experiences can overwhelm an individual's ability to cope, leading to a wide range of emotional, cognitive, and behavioral symptoms. These disorders are often triggered by direct exposure to trauma or by witnessing traumatic events.

Below are several significant disorders associated with trauma and stress:

Post-Traumatic Stress Disorder (PTSD): PTSD is one of the most well-known trauma-related disorders. It develops in response to a traumatic event, such as combat exposure, physical or sexual assault, natural disasters, accidents, or witnessing violence. Symptoms include intrusive memories, flashbacks, nightmares, hypervigilance, avoidance of reminders of the trauma, negative changes in mood and cognition, and heightened reactivity.

Acute Stress Disorder (ASD): ASD is similar to PTSD but occurs within a month of exposure to a traumatic event and lasts for a minimum of three days and up to four weeks. Symptoms may include intrusive memories, dissociative experiences, avoidance, negative mood, and changes in arousal and reactivity.

Adjustment Disorders: This category includes maladaptive emotional or behavioral reactions to identifiable stressors. While not necessarily caused by a traumatic event, these stressors can lead to significant distress and impairment. Symptoms might include anxiety, depression, impaired social or occupational functioning, or behavioral disturbances.

Reactive Attachment Disorder (RAD): RAD typically occurs in children who have experienced neglect, abuse, or disruptions in their early caregiving relationships. It involves difficulties forming healthy attachments to caregivers, leading to problems in emotional and social development.

Disinhibited Social Engagement Disorder: This disorder also often arises in children who have experienced neglect or disruptions in caregiving. Children with disinhibited social engagement disorder display overly familiar behavior with unfamiliar adults and a lack of appropriate fear or caution in social interactions.

Other Specified Trauma- and Stressor-Related Disorder and Unspecified Trauma- and Stressor-Related Disorder: These categories encompass conditions that do not fully meet the criteria for the specific disorders mentioned above but are still related to exposure to traumatic or stressful events.

These disorders can have a significant impact on an individual's emotional well-being, relationships, work, and daily functioning. They often result from a complex interplay of genetic, biological, environmental, and psychological factors.

Treatment for Trauma- and Stressor-Related Disorders typically involves various therapeutic approaches:

Psychotherapy: Trauma-focused therapies, such as cognitive-behavioral therapy (CBT), eye movement desensitization and reprocessing (EMDR), and exposure therapy, are often used to help individuals process traumatic experiences and manage symptoms.

Medication: In some cases, medications, such as antidepressants or anti-anxiety medications, may be prescribed to alleviate symptoms like anxiety, depression, or sleep disturbances.

Supportive Interventions: Support groups, stress management techniques, and interventions aimed at improving coping skills can be beneficial.

♦Early intervention and appropriate support are crucial in addressing Trauma- and Stressor-Related Disorders. Seeking help from mental health professionals who specialize in trauma can significantly aid in recovery and improve overall well-being.

Chapter 5

Dermatological Conditions

Dermatological conditions refer to a wide range of disorders and diseases that affect the skin, hair, nails, and mucous membranes. These conditions can be caused by various factors, including genetics, infections, immune system problems, environmental factors, and lifestyle choices. Dermatologists are medical professionals specialized in diagnosing and treating these conditions.

Some common dermatological conditions:

Eczema (Dermatitis): An inflammatory skin condition that causes redness, itching, and sometimes blistering. There are several types of eczema, with atopic dermatitis being the most common.

Skin Cancer: Various forms of skin cancer, including basal cell carcinoma, squamous cell carcinoma, and melanoma, are caused by the abnormal growth of skin cells due to damage from ultraviolet (UV) radiation.

Hives (Urticaria): Raised, itchy welts on the skin caused by an allergic reaction or other triggers. Hives can be acute or chronic.

Rosacea: A chronic skin condition that primarily affects the face, causing redness, flushing, visible blood vessels, and sometimes pimples and eye irritation.

Vitiligo: A condition in which the immune system attacks and destroys the melanocytes (pigment-producing cells), causing white patches on the skin.

Acne: A skin condition characterized by the formation of pimples, blackheads, whiteheads, and cysts, usually associated with increased oil production, bacteria, and inflammation.

Impetigo: A contagious bacterial infection that results in red sores and blisters, often around the mouth and nose, and is common in children.

♦It's important to note that proper diagnosis and treatment of dermatological conditions often require consultation with a healthcare professional, preferably a dermatologist. Additionally, some conditions may have systemic implications, affecting other organs and requiring a holistic approach to management. Regular skin examinations and sun protection are essential for maintaining skin health and preventing certain skin conditions.

Eczema (Dermatitis)

Eczema, also known as **dermatitis**, is a chronic inflammatory skin condition characterized by red, itchy, and inflamed skin. It is a common condition that can affect people of all ages, from infants to adults. Eczema is not contagious, and while it may be chronic, symptoms can often be managed with appropriate treatment.

Types of Eczema

Seborrheic Dermatitis: Often affects the scalp and face, causing redness, scaling, and dandruff.

Symptoms:

Itching: Intense itching is a hallmark symptom of eczema and can be severe, leading to scratching that worsens the condition.

Redness: The affected skin often becomes red or inflamed.

Dryness: Eczema-prone skin tends to be dry and may crack or peel.

Rash: Eczema can cause the development of a rash, which may vary in appearance depending on the type of eczema.

Causes and Triggers

•Genetics: Family history of eczema, asthma, or hay fever may increase the risk.

•Environmental Factors: Irritants such as soaps, detergents, and certain fabrics can trigger eczema.

•Allergens: Exposure to allergens like pollen, pet dander, or certain foods may exacerbate symptoms.

•Stress: Emotional stress can trigger or worsen eczema.

Diagnosis

Diagnosing eczema typically involves a thorough examination of the skin, a review of medical history, and, in some cases, allergy testing.

Treatment and Management

•Topical Steroids: These are often prescribed to reduce inflammation and itching.

•Topical Calcineurin Inhibitors: These medications, such as tacrolimus and pimecrolimus, can be used for certain types of eczema and are particularly helpful on the face.

Moisturizers: Regular use of emollients to keep the skin hydrated and prevent dryness.

•Avoiding Triggers: Identifying and avoiding substances or conditions that trigger eczema flares.

•Antihistamines: These may be recommended to help control itching, especially at night.

√Phototherapy: Controlled exposure to ultraviolet light under medical supervision.

Preventive Measures

•Gentle Skincare: Use mild soaps, avoid harsh •cleansers, and pat the skin dry rather than rubbing.

•Avoiding Irritants: Identify and minimize exposure to irritants and allergens.

•Cotton Clothing: Wear soft, breathable fabrics like cotton to reduce skin irritation.

•Stress Management: Stress reduction techniques can be beneficial in managing eczema.

Skin Cancer

Skin cancer is a type of cancer that develops in the skin cells. It is the most common form of cancer globally, and its incidence is primarily linked to exposure to ultraviolet (UV) radiation from the sun or artificial sources (such as tanning beds). There are different types of skin cancer, and they can vary in terms of severity and treatment. The three main types are **basal cell carcinoma (BCC), squamous cell carcinoma (SCC), and melanoma**.

Basal Cell Carcinoma (BCC):

•Characteristics: BCC is the most common type of skin cancer, and it usually appears on areas of the skin that are frequently exposed to the sun, such as the face and neck.
•Appearance: BCC often presents as a pearly or waxy bump, a flat, flesh-colored or brown scar-like lesion, or a bleeding or oozing sore that doesn't heal.
Squamous Cell Carcinoma (SCC):

•Characteristics: SCC is the second most common type of skin cancer. It is more likely to spread than BCC, although it usually remains localized.
•Appearance: SCC often appears as a red nodule or a flat, scaly, crusty lesion, and it may bleed easily.
Melanoma:

•Characteristics: Melanoma is less common but more aggressive than BCC and SCC. It develops in the cells that produce melanin, the pigment responsible for skin color.
•Appearance: Melanomas are often characterized by an irregularly shaped and colored mole. They may be asymmetrical, have uneven borders, exhibit variations in color (shades of brown, black, or even red and blue), have a diameter larger than a pencil eraser, and may evolve or change over time.

Risk Factors

•UV Radiation: Overexposure to UV radiation from the sun or tanning beds is a major risk factor.
•Fair Skin: People with fair skin, light hair, and light-colored eyes are at higher risk.
•Family History: A family history of skin cancer can increase the risk.
•Weakened Immune System: Individuals with weakened immune systems are at higher risk.

Prevention:

•Sun Protection: Wearing protective clothing, using sunscreen with a high SPF, and avoiding peak sun hours can reduce the risk of skin cancer.
Regular Skin Checks: Self-examinations and regular professional skin checks are important for early detection.

Diagnosis

Dermatologists typically diagnose skin cancer through visual examination, and they may perform a biopsy for confirmation.

Treatment

•Surgery: Surgical removal is the primary treatment for most skin cancers.
√Mohs Surgery: This technique involves removing thin layers of cancer-containing skin until only cancer-free tissue remains.
•Radiation Therapy: It may be used for certain cases where surgery is not suitable.
•Chemotherapy or Immunotherapy: These systemic treatments may be recommended for advanced cases, especially for melanoma.

♦Early detection and treatment significantly improve the outcomes of skin cancer. Regular skin examinations and self-checks are crucial for identifying any changes in moles or the appearance of new lesions. Individuals are advised to consult with a healthcare professional, especially a dermatologist, for personalized advice and monitoring.

Hives (Urticaria)

Hives, medically termed urticaria, is a skin condition characterized by the sudden appearance of raised, red, itchy welts or wheals on the skin. These welts can vary in size, shape, and location and often occur in clusters. Hives can be acute, lasting less than six weeks, or chronic, lasting more than six weeks.

Key Features of Hives (Urticaria):

Appearance

Hives typically present as raised, red or pink welts on the skin. The borders may be well-defined or irregular.

The welts are often intensely itchy and may appear suddenly and disappear within hours, only to reappear elsewhere on the body.

Duration

•Acute Hives: These can appear suddenly and often resolve on their own within a few hours to days. Common triggers include certain foods, medications, insect stings, infections, or exposure to allergens.

•Chronic Hives: When hives persist for more than six weeks, it is considered chronic. Identifying the cause of chronic hives can be more challenging, and it may be related to underlying health conditions.

Causes and Triggers

•Allergic Reactions: Hives can be triggered by allergies to foods (such as nuts, shellfish), medications (like antibiotics), insect stings, or latex.

•Non-Allergic Causes: Some cases of hives are not related to allergies and can be triggered by factors like stress, infections, changes in temperature, pressure on the skin (dermatographism), or certain illnesses.

Underlying Conditions:

Chronic hives may be associated with underlying conditions such as autoimmune disorders, thyroid dysfunction, or chronic infections.

Diagnosis

Diagnosis is often based on a thorough medical history and physical examination.

In some cases, additional tests may be performed to identify the underlying cause, especially for chronic hives.

Treatment

•Antihistamines: These are the primary medications used to relieve itching and reduce the severity of hives.

•Corticosteroids: In severe cases, short-term use of oral corticosteroids may be prescribed.

Identifying and Avoiding Triggers: For hives triggered by allergies, identifying and avoiding the specific allergen is crucial.

•Immune Modulators: In some cases, medications that modulate the immune system may be prescribed for chronic hives.

Management and Prevention:

•Avoiding Triggers: Identifying and avoiding triggers, when possible, can help prevent the recurrence of hives.

•Maintaining a Symptom Diary: Keeping a record of activities, foods, and exposures can assist in identifying potential triggers.

•Stress Management: Stress reduction techniques may be beneficial for individuals with stress-induced hives.

Emergency Situations

In rare cases, hives can be accompanied by severe swelling, difficulty breathing, or other symptoms indicative of a severe allergic reaction (anaphylaxis). This requires immediate medical attention.

It's important for individuals experiencing hives to consult with a healthcare professional, especially a dermatologist or allergist, for proper diagnosis and management. Chronic cases may require a more comprehensive evaluation to identify any underlying health conditions.

Rosacea

Rosacea is a common and chronic skin condition that primarily affects the face. It often begins with a tendency to blush or flush more easily than other people, and over time, it can progress to persistent redness, visible blood vessels, and other symptoms. Rosacea tends to affect fair-skinned individuals, particularly those of Northern European descent, and it is more common in women.

Features of Rosacea

Facial Redness (Erythema):

Persistent redness on the central part of the face, including the forehead, nose, cheeks, and chin.
The redness may come and go but can become more pronounced over time.

Flushing and Blushing:

Individuals with rosacea often experience episodes of flushing or blushing more easily than others.
Triggers for flushing can include exposure to sunlight, hot drinks, spicy foods, alcohol, and emotional stress.

Visible Blood Vessels (Telangiectasia):

Small blood vessels (capillaries) near the surface of the skin become visible, giving the appearance of fine red lines.

Papules and **Pustules**

Inflammatory bumps resembling acne may develop. These can be papules (small, red, solid bumps) or pustules (pus-filled bumps).
Unlike acne, there are usually no blackheads, and the lesions are often not as painful.

Phymatous Changes:
In some cases, especially if left untreated, rosacea can lead to thickening of the skin, particularly on the nose (rhinophyma) or other facial areas. This is more common in men.

Ocular Symptoms

Some individuals with rosacea may experience eye-related symptoms, including redness, dryness, burning, and sensitivity to light (ocular rosacea).

Triggers

Rosacea symptoms can be triggered or exacerbated by various factors, including sunlight, hot or spicy foods, alcohol, stress, and certain medications.
Subtypes of Rosacea:

Erythematotelangiectatic Rosacea (ETR): Characterized by persistent facial redness and visible blood vessels.
Papulopustular Rosacea: Involves papules and pustules in addition to redness.
Phymatous Rosacea: Involves thickening of the skin, particularly on the nose.
Ocular Rosacea: Involves eye-related symptoms.
Diagnosis:

A dermatologist typically diagnoses rosacea based on the characteristic symptoms and appearance of the skin. There is no specific test for rosacea.

Treatment

•Topical Medications: Prescription creams or gels containing metronidazole, azelaic acid, or other ingredients may be used to reduce inflammation.

•Oral Antibiotics: In some cases, oral antibiotics, such as tetracycline or doxycycline, may be prescribed to control inflammation.

•Laser Therapy: For visible blood vessels or redness, laser or intense pulsed light (IPL) therapy may be used.

•Topical Brimonidine: A medication that can temporarily reduce facial redness.

Management

•Identifying Triggers: Avoiding triggers that worsen symptoms.

•Gentle Skincare: Using mild, non-irritating skin care products.

•Sun Protection: Regular use of sunscreen to protect the skin from UV rays.

♦While rosacea is a chronic condition, proper management and treatment can control symptoms and improve the quality of life for individuals with this skin condition. Consulting with a dermatologist is essential for an accurate diagnosis and personalized treatment plan.

<u>Vitiligo</u>

Vitiligo is a chronic skin condition characterized by the loss of pigment in certain areas of the skin, resulting in white patches. This occurs due to the destruction of melanocytes, the cells responsible for producing the pigment melanin. Melanin gives color to the skin, hair, and eyes, and its absence in affected areas leads to the development of depigmented patches.

Symptoms

The primary symptom of vitiligo is the presence of depigmented or white patches on the skin.

These patches can vary in size and shape and may be surrounded by areas of normal pigmentation.

Vitiligo can affect any part of the body, including the face, hands, feet, elbows, knees, and genitalia.

Causes

The exact cause of vitiligo is not fully understood, but it is believed to involve a combination of genetic, autoimmune, and environmental factors.

Autoimmune theory suggests that the body's immune system mistakenly attacks and destroys its own melanocytes.

Risk Factors:

•Family History: Having a family member with vitiligo increases the risk.

•Autoimmune Diseases: Individuals with other autoimmune conditions, such as thyroid disorders or diabetes, may have a higher risk.

•Environmental Factors: Certain environmental triggers, such as exposure to chemicals or stress, may contribute.

Types of Vitiligo:

•Non-Segmental (Generalized) Vitiligo: The most common type, characterized by widespread and symmetrical depigmentation.

•Segmental Vitiligo: Involves depigmentation on one side or segment of the body and tends to progress for a limited period.

Diagnosis

Diagnosis is usually based on a visual examination of the skin and medical history.

In some cases, a skin biopsy may be performed to confirm the absence of melanocytes.

Treatment

While there is no cure for vitiligo, various treatment options aim to restore color to the affected skin or even out skin tone. Treatment effectiveness can vary among individuals.

•Topical Corticosteroids: These may be applied to the affected areas to reduce inflammation and promote repigmentation.

•Topical Calcineurin Inhibitors: Similar to their use in eczema, these medications can be used to suppress the immune response in the affected skin.

•Phototherapy (Light Therapy): Exposure to ultraviolet A (UVA) or ultraviolet B (UVB) light under controlled conditions can stimulate repigmentation.

•Depigmentation: In cases where vitiligo affects a large portion of the body, depigmentation of the remaining normal skin may be an option.

•Emotional and Psychological Impact:

The cosmetic impact of vitiligo can lead to emotional and psychological challenges, including social stigma and a negative impact on self-esteem. Support groups and counseling can be valuable for individuals coping with the emotional aspects of vitiligo.

♦It's important for individuals with vitiligo to consult with a dermatologist to discuss treatment options, manage expectations, and address any emotional or psychological concerns. Ongoing research is focused on understanding the underlying causes of vitiligo and developing more effective treatments.

Acne

Acne is a common skin condition that occurs when hair follicles become clogged with oil, dead skin cells, and bacteria. It often presents as pimples, blackheads, whiteheads, and, in more severe cases, cysts or nodules. Acne can affect various parts of the body, but it is most commonly found on the face, chest, back, and shoulders.

Let's break down the key aspects of Acne.

Hair Follicles and Sebaceous Glands:

Acne usually begins in hair follicles, which are small cavities in the skin from which hairs grow. Surrounding these follicles are sebaceous glands that produce an oily substance called sebum.

Excess Sebum Production:

Hormonal changes, especially during puberty, can stimulate the sebaceous glands to produce more sebum.

Excess sebum can mix with dead skin cells, leading to the formation of a plug in the hair follicles.

Formation of Comedones:

When the hair follicle becomes plugged, it can result in the formation of different types of lesions:

•**Blackheads (Open Comedones):** The plugged follicle is open at the skin's surface, and the material inside oxidizes, turning black.

•**Whiteheads (Closed Comedones):** The plugged follicle is closed, and the material inside does not oxidize. It appears as a white bump beneath the skin.

Proliferation of Bacteria:

Propionibacterium acnes, a bacterium that normally lives on the skin, can multiply in the plugged hair follicles.

The presence of bacteria can trigger inflammation and the formation of red, swollen lesions.

Inflammation and **Types of Acne Lesions:**

•Papules: Small, red, raised bumps caused by inflammation.

•Pustules: Pimples containing pus at their tips.

•Nodules: Large, painful, solid lesions beneath the skin's surface.

•Cysts: Painful, pus-filled lesions deeper in the skin, often leading to scarring.

Factors Contributing to Acne:

•Hormonal Changes: Common during puberty, menstruation, pregnancy, and certain medical conditions.

•Genetics: A family history of acne can increase the likelihood of developing the condition.

•Diet: While the impact of diet on acne is not fully understood, some studies suggest a link between high glycemic index foods and dairy with acne.

Treatment Options

•Topical Treatments: Include over-the-counter or prescription creams, gels, or lotions containing ingredients like benzoyl peroxide, salicylic acid, or retinoids.

•Oral Medications: Antibiotics, oral contraceptives (for females), and isotretinoin (a potent retinoid) may be prescribed in more severe cases.

•Procedures: Dermatological procedures such as chemical peels, laser therapy, or drainage and extraction may be considered for certain types of acne or scarring.

Preventive Measures

•Good Skin Hygiene: Regular cleansing to remove excess oil and dead skin cells.

•Avoiding Squeezing or Picking: This can worsen inflammation and increase the risk of scarring.

•Sun Protection: Some acne medications can increase sensitivity to sunlight, making sun protection important.

◆It's important to consult with a healthcare professional or dermatologist for an accurate diagnosis and personalized treatment plan based on the severity and type of acne. Early intervention and consistent management can help minimize the risk of scarring and improve the overall outcome.

Impetigo

Impetigo is a highly contagious bacterial skin infection that primarily affects children, but it can also occur in adults. It's caused by either Staphylococcus aureus or Streptococcus pyogenes bacteria and typically develops on areas where the skin has been damaged by cuts, scrapes, or insect bites.

Types of Impetigo

•Nonbullous Impetigo: This is the most common form, characterized by red sores that quickly rupture, ooze, and form a yellowish-brown crust.
•Bullous Impetigo: Less common, characterized by larger blisters that contain clear fluid and eventually burst, leaving a yellow crust.

Symptoms

Red sores or blisters that rupture and ooze fluid.

Formation of honey-colored crusts over the affected area.

Itching and discomfort around the affected skin.

Transmission

Impetigo is highly contagious and spreads through direct contact with the sores or by touching contaminated objects.

It can also spread from one part of the body to another through scratching or touching.

Risk Factors

Children, particularly those aged 2 to 5, are more susceptible due to their close contact in schools or daycare settings.

Warm and humid climates may also increase the risk.

Diagnosis

Usually diagnosed based on the appearance of the sores and crusts. A swab or culture of the affected area may be taken to identify the specific bacteria causing the infection.

Treatment

•Topical Antibiotics: Antibiotic ointments or creams are often prescribed to apply to the affected area.

•Oral Antibiotics: In more severe cases or when the infection spreads, oral antibiotics may be necessary. Keeping the affected area clean and covered with gauze to prevent the spread of infection.

Preventive Measures:

Practice good hygiene, including regular handwashing.

Keep cuts, scrapes, and other skin injuries clean and covered.

Avoid sharing personal items like towels or clothing with infected individuals.

Complications:

In some cases, impetigo can lead to more serious complications, such as cellulitis (a deeper skin infection) or poststreptococcal glomerulonephritis (a kidney condition).

Healing and Contagiousness:

With treatment, impetigo usually clears up within a week or so.

Individuals with impetigo should avoid close contact with others until the sores have crusted over and healed to prevent spreading the infection.

Medical Advice

♦It's important to consult a healthcare professional, such as a doctor or dermatologist, for proper diagnosis and treatment, especially if the infection worsens or spreads.

Early treatment of impetigo helps reduce the risk of complications and prevents its spread to others. Practicing good hygiene habits and prompt treatment of any skin injuries can help prevent impetigo.

Chapter 6
Endocrine conditions

Endocrine conditions refer to disorders or diseases that affect the endocrine system, which is a complex network of glands that produce and release hormones into the bloodstream. These hormones play a crucial role in regulating various physiological processes and maintaining overall balance within the body. The endocrine system includes glands such as the pituitary, thyroid, adrenal, pancreas, ovaries, and testes.

Common endocrine conditions are:

Hypothyroidism:Insufficient production of thyroid hormones by the thyroid gland.
Hyperthyroidism:Overproduction of thyroid hormones by the thyroid gland.
Hyperaldosteronism:Description: Overproduction of aldosterone by the adrenal glands.
Hyperparathyroidism:Description: Overproduction of parathyroid hormone.
Addison's Disease:Description: Insufficient production of cortisol and aldosterone by the adrenal glands.

Diabetes Mellitus: A group of metabolic disorders characterized by high blood sugar levels resulting from inadequate insulin production or the body's inability to use insulin effectively.

Hypothyroidism

Hypothyroidism is a medical condition characterized by an underactive thyroid gland, which means the thyroid gland doesn't produce enough thyroid hormones to meet the body's needs. The thyroid hormones, primarily thyroxine (T4) and triiodothyronine (T3), play a crucial role in regulating metabolism and energy production in the body. When their levels are insufficient, various bodily functions slow down, leading to a range of symptoms.

Causes

•Autoimmune Thyroiditis (Hashimoto's Thyroiditis): The most common cause of hypothyroidism is an autoimmune condition where the body's immune system mistakenly attacks and damages the thyroid gland, reducing its ability to produce hormones.

•Iodine Deficiency: The thyroid gland requires iodine to produce thyroid hormones. Insufficient iodine in the diet can lead to hypothyroidism.

•Thyroid Surgery or Radiation Therapy: Removal of the thyroid gland or exposure to radiation around the neck area can result in decreased hormone production.

•Certain Medications: Some medications, such as lithium or certain anti-thyroid drugs, can interfere with thyroid hormone production.

•Congenital Hypothyroidism: Some individuals are born with an underactive thyroid gland due to a congenital defect.

Symptoms

•Fatigue: Individuals with hypothyroidism often experience persistent tiredness and a lack of energy.
•Weight Gain: Slowed metabolism can lead to weight gain, even with reduced food intake.
•Cold Sensitivity: A feeling of being excessively sensitive to cold temperatures.
•Dry Skin and Hair: Skin and hair may become dry and brittle.
•Constipation: Reduced activity in the digestive system can lead to constipation.

•Muscle Weakness and Joint Pain: Weakness in the muscles and pain in the joints.

•Depression and Cognitive Issues: Hypothyroidism can affect mood and cognitive function, leading to depression, forgetfulness, and difficulty concentrating.

•Menstrual Irregularities: Women with hypothyroidism may experience irregular menstrual cycles.

•Elevated Cholesterol Levels: Hypothyroidism can contribute to higher levels of cholesterol in the blood.

Diagnosis and Treatment

Diagnosis is typically based on a combination of symptoms, physical examination, and blood tests measuring levels of thyroid hormones (T3 and T4) and thyroid-stimulating hormone (TSH). Treatment usually involves thyroid hormone replacement therapy, where synthetic thyroid hormones (levothyroxine) are prescribed to supplement the deficient hormones. The goal is to bring thyroid hormone levels back to normal, alleviating symptoms and restoring normal metabolic function.

♦It's important for individuals with hypothyroidism to undergo regular monitoring and adjustment of medication dosage as needed. With proper treatment, most people with hypothyroidism can lead normal, healthy lives. It's crucial for individuals experiencing symptoms suggestive of hypothyroidism to consult with a healthcare professional for a proper diagnosis and appropriate management.

Hyperthyroidism

Hyperthyroidism is a medical condition characterized by an overactive thyroid gland, leading to an excessive production of thyroid hormones—thyroxine (T4) and triiodothyronine (T3). These hormones play a crucial role in regulating the body's metabolism, and when their levels are elevated, various bodily functions speed up, causing a range of symptoms. **It's the opposite of hypothyroidism.**

Causes

•Graves' Disease: The most common cause of hyperthyroidism, Graves' disease is an autoimmune disorder where the immune system stimulates the thyroid to produce too much thyroid hormone.

•Toxic Nodular Goiter: The thyroid gland develops nodules that produce thyroid hormones independently of the body's regulatory mechanisms.

•Subacute Thyroiditis: Inflammation of the thyroid gland, often triggered by a viral infection, can cause a temporary increase in thyroid hormone levels.

•Excessive Iodine Intake: Consuming too much iodine, either through diet or medications, can lead to hyperthyroidism.

•Thyroiditis: Inflammation of the thyroid gland can cause a temporary release of stored hormones into the bloodstream.

•Tumors: Benign or malignant tumors of the thyroid or pituitary gland can lead to hyperthyroidism.

Symptoms

•Weight Loss: Despite an increased appetite, individuals with hyperthyroidism may lose weight.

•Increased Heart Rate: A rapid or irregular heartbeat (palpitations) is common.

•Nervousness and Anxiety: Hyperthyroidism can lead to heightened levels of anxiety and nervousness.

•Tremors: Fine tremors, especially in the hands, may occur.

•Heat Intolerance: Individuals may feel excessively warm and sweat more than usual.

•Fatigue: Paradoxically, some individuals with hyperthyroidism may also experience fatigue.

•Muscle Weakness: Weakness and fatigue in the muscles.

•Difficulty Sleeping: Insomnia or difficulty sleeping can be a symptom.

•Changes in Menstrual Patterns: Women may experience irregular menstrual cycles.

•Enlarged Thyroid (Goiter): The thyroid gland may become visibly enlarged.

Diagnosis and Treatment

Diagnosis typically involves blood tests to measure levels of T3, T4, and thyroid-stimulating hormone (TSH). Imaging studies, such as thyroid scans, may also be performed to identify the underlying cause. Once diagnosed, the goal of treatment is to reduce

the production of thyroid hormones and manage symptoms.
Treatment options include:

•Antithyroid Medications: Drugs like methimazole and propylthiouracil can inhibit the production of thyroid hormones.

•Radioactive Iodine Therapy: Radioactive iodine is taken orally, and it selectively destroys the overactive thyroid cells.

•Beta-Blockers: These medications help manage symptoms such as rapid heart rate and tremors.

•Thyroidectomy: Surgical removal of part or all of the thyroid gland may be recommended in certain cases.

♦Effective management of hyperthyroidism usually requires ongoing medical supervision to monitor hormone levels and adjust treatment as needed. If left untreated, hyperthyroidism can lead to complications such as heart problems, osteoporosis, and other health issues. Therefore, seeking medical attention for proper diagnosis and treatment is essential for individuals experiencing symptoms suggestive of hyperthyroidism.

Hyperaldosteronism

Hyperaldosteronism is a medical condition characterized by the overproduction of aldosterone, a hormone produced by the adrenal glands. Aldosterone plays a key role in regulating the balance of sodium and potassium in the body, which in turn influences blood pressure and fluid balance. When there is an excessive production of aldosterone, it can lead to disruptions in these balances, resulting in various symptoms and potential complications.

Types of Hyperaldosteronism:
Primary Hyperaldosteronism (Conn's Syndrome):

This occurs when there is an issue with the adrenal glands themselves, leading to overproduction of aldosterone. The most common cause is typically an adrenal adenoma (a benign tumor) or, less commonly, adrenal hyperplasia (enlargement).
Secondary Hyperaldosteronism:

This is usually a response to an outside stimulus that prompts the adrenal glands to produce more aldosterone. Common causes include kidney disease, heart failure, or conditions that cause low blood flow to the kidneys.

Symptoms of Hyperaldosteronism:

•Hypertension (High Blood Pressure):

Persistent high blood pressure that may be difficult to control with standard medications.

•Hypokalemia:

Low levels of potassium in the blood, which can lead to weakness, muscle cramps, and irregular heart rhythms.

•Muscle Weakness:

Generalized weakness and fatigue.

•Frequent Urination:

Increased urination and thirst.

•Headache:

Persistent or severe headaches may occur.

•Alkalosis:

Elevated blood pH due to increased excretion of hydrogen ions in the urine.

Diagnosis and Treatment

•Blood Tests:

Measurement of aldosterone levels and the aldosterone-to-renin ratio helps in diagnosis.

•Imaging Studies:

CT scans or MRI may be used to identify abnormalities in the adrenal glands.

•Adrenal Vein Sampling:

In some cases, a specialized test involving sampling blood from the adrenal veins may be conducted to identify which adrenal gland is producing excess aldosterone.

Treatment options depend on the underlying cause:

•Primary Hyperaldosteronism (Conn's Syndrome):

Surgical removal of the affected adrenal gland (adrenalectomy) is often the preferred treatment, especially if there is a benign tumor (adenoma).
•Secondary Hyperaldosteronism:

Treatment involves addressing the underlying cause, such as managing kidney disease or heart failure.
In some cases, medications may be prescribed to manage blood pressure and correct potassium imbalances. Medications like aldosterone antagonists may be used to block the effects of excess aldosterone.

♦Regular monitoring of blood pressure, electrolyte levels, and kidney function is crucial for individuals with hyperaldosteronism. Early diagnosis and appropriate management can help prevent complications related to hypertension and electrolyte imbalances.

Addison's disease

Addison's disease, also known as primary adrenal insufficiency, is a rare but serious disorder characterized by the insufficient production of adrenal hormones by the adrenal glands. The adrenal glands are small, triangular-shaped glands located on top of each kidney. They produce essential hormones, including cortisol and aldosterone, that play crucial roles in regulating various bodily functions.

Causes of Addison's Disease:
The most common cause of Addison's disease is **autoimmune adrenalitis**, where the body's immune system mistakenly attacks and damages the adrenal glands. Other causes may include:

•Infections: Tuberculosis and certain fungal infections can affect the adrenal glands.

•Cancer: Tumors in the adrenal glands can impair hormone production.

•Genetic Factors: In rare cases, Addison's disease can be inherited.

•Certain Medications: Long-term use of medications like glucocorticoids can suppress adrenal function.

Symptoms of Addison's Disease:
The symptoms of Addison's disease often develop gradually and may include:
•Fatigue: Persistent and overwhelming tiredness.
•Weight Loss: Unintentional weight loss.
•Low Blood Pressure: Hypotension, which can lead to dizziness and fainting.
•Hyperpigmentation: Darkening of the skin, particularly in sun-exposed areas and skin creases.
•Salt Cravings: Due to low aldosterone levels, individuals may crave salty foods.
•Hypoglycemia: Low blood sugar levels, leading to weakness and shakiness.
•Nausea and Vomiting: Gastrointestinal symptoms can occur.
•Muscle or Joint Pain: Weakness, pain, and muscle aches.
•Mood Changes: Irritability and depression.
•Menstrual Irregularities: In women, menstrual periods may become irregular or stop.

Diagnosis and Treatment:
Diagnosis involves a combination of clinical evaluation, blood tests measuring cortisol and

aldosterone levels, and, in some cases, stimulation tests to assess the adrenal glands' response to specific hormones.

Treatment for Addison's disease typically involves lifelong hormone replacement therapy to replace the deficient hormones. The two main types of hormones replaced are:

Glucocorticoids (usually hydrocortisone): These hormones help regulate metabolism and the body's response to stress.

Mineralocorticoids (usually fludrocortisone): These hormones help maintain the balance of salt and water in the body.

Patients with Addison's disease need to take these medications regularly and adjust their dosage during times of stress, such as illness or surgery. Regular medical follow-up is essential to monitor hormone levels and adjust treatment as needed.

♦If left untreated or inadequately managed, Addison's disease can lead to a life-threatening condition called an adrenal crisis, characterized by severe symptoms such as low blood pressure, confusion, and even loss of consciousness. Therefore, prompt diagnosis and appropriate medical management are crucial for individuals with Addison's disease.

<u>Diabetes mellitus</u>

Diabetes mellitus refers to a group of metabolic disorders characterized by high blood sugar levels (hyperglycemia) over an extended period. The condition arises due to either insufficient insulin production by the pancreas or the body's ineffective use of insulin, or a combination of both factors. Insulin, a hormone produced by the pancreas, helps regulate blood sugar levels by facilitating the uptake of glucose from the bloodstream into cells for energy or storage.

Types of Diabetes Mellitus
•**Type 1 Diabetes:**
Occurs when the immune system mistakenly attacks and destroys insulin-producing beta cells in the pancreas. This leads to little to no insulin production.
Typically diagnosed in childhood or adolescence, but can develop at any age.
Management involves insulin therapy.
•**Type 2 Diabetes:**

Results from insulin resistance, where cells do not respond effectively to insulin, or insufficient insulin production.

Often associated with lifestyle factors such as obesity, sedentary lifestyle, and genetic predisposition.

Initially managed with lifestyle changes (diet, exercise) and medications. Some individuals may require insulin therapy.

•**Gestational Diabetes**:

Occurs during pregnancy and usually resolves after childbirth. It can increase the risk of complications for both the mother and baby.

Managed with dietary changes, exercise, and sometimes insulin therapy.

Symptoms of Diabetes Mellitus:

•**Polyuria:**

Excessive urination due to the body's attempt to eliminate excess glucose through urine.

•**Polydipsia:**

Increased thirst, as a response to dehydration caused by excessive urination.

•**Polyphagia:**

Increased hunger and food intake, as cells are deprived of energy despite high blood sugar levels.

•**Weight Loss:**

Unintended weight loss, particularly in Type 1 diabetes, due to the body breaking down muscle and fat for energy.

•Fatigue:
Generalized tiredness and lack of energy.
•Blurred Vision:
Changes in vision due to fluctuations in blood sugar levels.

Diagnosis and Treatment

Diagnosis involves blood tests measuring fasting blood sugar levels, oral glucose tolerance tests, or glycated hemoglobin (HbA1c) levels, which reflect average blood sugar levels over the past few months.

Treatment aims to control blood sugar levels and prevent complications. It often includes:

•Lifestyle Modifications:
Healthy diet, regular exercise, weight management.
•Medications:
Oral medications to lower blood sugar or insulin injections to replace or supplement natural insulin.
•Monitoring:
Regular monitoring of blood sugar levels to track control and adjust treatment as needed.
Complications of uncontrolled diabetes include cardiovascular diseases, kidney damage, nerve damage, vision impairment, and foot problems. Therefore, proper management and regular medical care are crucial to prevent complications and maintain overall health for individuals with diabetes mellitus.

Chapter 7

Hematological conditions

Hematological conditions refer to disorders or diseases that affect the blood and its components, including blood cells (red blood cells, white blood cells, and platelets) and the plasma. These conditions can arise from various causes, including genetic factors, infections, autoimmune reactions, nutritional deficiencies, and environmental factors.

Examples hematological conditions

Anemia:

Anemia is a condition characterized by a decrease in the number of red blood cells or a deficiency of hemoglobin, the oxygen-carrying protein in red blood cells. This can result in fatigue, weakness, and pale skin.

Hemophilia:

Hemophilia is a genetic disorder that impairs the blood's ability to clot. People with hemophilia may experience prolonged bleeding after injuries or surgery.

Leukemia:

Leukemia is a type of cancer that affects the blood and bone marrow. It results in the uncontrolled production of abnormal white blood cells, which can crowd out normal cells and affect the body's ability to fight infections.

Lymphoma:

Lymphoma is a type of cancer that affects the lymphatic system, which is a part of the immune system. There are two main types: Hodgkin lymphoma and non-Hodgkin lymphoma.

Hemochromatosis:

Hemochromatosis is a condition where the body absorbs too much iron from the diet, leading to an excess of iron in the organs. Over time, this can damage the liver, heart, and other organs.

Diagnosis and treatment of hematological conditions often involve blood tests, bone marrow biopsies, and various medical interventions such as blood transfusions, medications, chemotherapy, or bone marrow transplantation, depending on the specific condition and its severity. It's important for individuals with symptoms or risk factors for hematological conditions to seek medical attention for proper diagnosis and management.

Anemia

Anemia is a medical condition characterized by a reduced number of red blood cells (RBCs) or a lower than normal concentration of hemoglobin in the blood. Hemoglobin is a protein present in red blood cells that binds to oxygen and carries it from the lungs to the rest of the body. Anemia can result in a decreased ability of the blood to carry oxygen to tissues and organs, leading to various symptoms.

There are several types and causes of anemia, each with its own characteristics.
Common types of anemia and their causes:

Iron-Deficiency Anemia:

This is the most common type of anemia. It occurs when the body doesn't have enough iron to produce sufficient hemoglobin. Causes can include inadequate dietary intake of iron, poor absorption of iron from the digestive tract, or chronic blood loss (e.g., from gastrointestinal bleeding or heavy menstrual periods).

Vitamin Deficiency Anemias:

Deficiencies in certain vitamins, such as vitamin B12 and folic acid (folate), can lead to anemia. These vitamins are essential for the production of healthy red blood cells. A lack of these vitamins may occur due to poor dietary intake, malabsorption issues, or other medical conditions.

Hemolytic Anemias:

Hemolytic anemias result from the destruction of red blood cells at a rate faster than the body can produce them. This can be due to genetic factors, autoimmune reactions, infections, or certain medications.

Aplastic Anemia:

Aplastic anemia is a rare condition where the bone marrow fails to produce an adequate number of blood cells, including red blood cells. It can be caused by genetic factors, exposure to certain toxins, or autoimmune disorders.

Chronic Diseases:

Some chronic diseases, such as chronic kidney disease, inflammatory disorders, or certain types of cancer, can lead to anemia due to various mechanisms, including reduced production of red blood cells or increased destruction.

Sickle Cell Anemia:

Sickle cell anemia is a genetic disorder where red blood cells have an abnormal, crescent shape. These

misshapen cells can break down more easily, leading to a chronic shortage of red blood cells.
Common symptoms of anemia include fatigue, weakness, pale or sallow skin, shortness of breath, dizziness, and cold hands and feet. The specific symptoms and severity can vary depending on the underlying cause and the degree of anemia.

Diagnosis typically involves blood tests to measure hemoglobin levels, red blood cell count, and other relevant parameters. Treatment aims to address the underlying cause and may include dietary changes, iron supplements, vitamin supplements, blood transfusions, or other interventions, depending on the specific type of anemia.

♦It's crucial for individuals experiencing symptoms of anemia to seek medical attention for proper diagnosis and treatment.

<u>Hemophilia</u>

Hemophilia is a genetic disorder that affects the blood's ability to clot properly. Individuals with hemophilia experience prolonged bleeding after injuries or surgery due to a deficiency or dysfunction of certain clotting factors in the blood.

There are two main types of hemophilia: hemophilia A and hemophilia B.

Hemophilia A:
Hemophilia A is the more common type, and it results from a deficiency or dysfunction of clotting factor VIII (factor eight).

Hemophilia B:
Hemophilia B is less common and is caused by a deficiency or dysfunction of clotting factor IX (factor nine).

Causes and Genetics

Hemophilia is an inherited disorder, meaning it is passed down through families. The condition is linked to the X chromosome. Since males have one X and one Y chromosome (XY), and females have two X chromosomes (XX), hemophilia is more common in males. Females are typically carriers of the gene but may not exhibit symptoms themselves.

If a woman carries the hemophilia gene, there is a 50% chance of passing it on to her children, regardless of their gender. If a man with hemophilia has children with a woman who is not a carrier, their daughters will be carriers, and their sons will not have hemophilia.

Symptoms

The severity of hemophilia can vary. Individuals with mild hemophilia may only bleed excessively after surgery or trauma, while those with severe hemophilia may experience spontaneous bleeding.

Common symptoms include:

•Excessive bleeding: Prolonged bleeding after cuts, injuries, or surgery.
•Joint and muscle bleeds: Bleeding into joints and muscles can cause pain, swelling, and limited range of motion.
•Spontaneous bleeding: Without an apparent cause, individuals may experience spontaneous bleeding, especially into joints.

Diagnosis and Treatment

Diagnosis involves blood tests to measure the levels of clotting factors. Prenatal testing is also available for families with a history of hemophilia.

Treatment typically involves replacement therapy to restore the missing clotting factor. This can be done on an as-needed basis (known as on-demand treatment) or as a preventive measure (known as prophylactic treatment) to reduce the risk of spontaneous bleeding. Clotting factor replacement can be derived from human blood products or produced synthetically.

Physical therapy may be recommended to manage joint problems, and medications may be used to alleviate pain and reduce inflammation associated with bleeding episodes.

Living with Hemophilia

♦While there is no cure for hemophilia, advances in treatment have significantly improved the quality of life for individuals with the condition. With appropriate medical care and precautions, individuals with hemophilia can lead active and fulfilling lives. It's essential for individuals with hemophilia to work closely with healthcare professionals to manage their condition and prevent complications.

Leukemia

Leukemia is a type of cancer that affects the blood and bone marrow. It is characterized by the uncontrolled production of abnormal white blood cells, which are crucial for the body's immune system. Leukemia can be acute or chronic, and there are several subtypes based on the specific type of white blood cell affected.

Types of Leukemia

•Acute Lymphoblastic Leukemia (ALL):

ALL is a type of leukemia that primarily affects lymphocytes, a type of white blood cell. It is more common in children, but it can also occur in adults.
•Chronic Lymphocytic Leukemia (CLL):

CLL is a slow-progressing leukemia that affects mature lymphocytes, and it is more common in adults, particularly those over the age of 60.
Acute Myeloid Leukemia (AML):

AML affects myeloid cells and is characterized by the rapid growth of abnormal white blood cells. It can occur in both children and adults.
•Chronic Myeloid Leukemia (CML):

CML is a slowly progressing leukemia that primarily affects myeloid cells. It often starts in the bone marrow and then progresses to the blood.
Causes and Risk Factors:
The exact cause of leukemia is often unknown, but several factors may increase the risk of developing the disease, including:

•Genetic Factors: Some genetic abnormalities are associated with an increased risk of leukemia.

•Radiation Exposure: Exposure to high levels of radiation, such as from certain medical treatments or nuclear accidents, may increase the risk.

•Chemical Exposure: Exposure to certain chemicals, such as benzene, has been linked to an increased risk.

•Certain Medical Conditions: Some genetic syndromes and pre-existing blood disorders may predispose individuals to leukemia.

Symptoms

The symptoms of leukemia can vary depending on the type and stage of the disease, but common signs may include:

•Fatigue
•Weakness
•Frequent infections
•Pale or sallow skin
•Easy bruising or bleeding
•Enlarged lymph nodes or spleen
•Unexplained weight loss

Diagnosis and Treatment

Diagnosis typically involves blood tests, bone marrow biopsy, and imaging studies. Treatment varies based on the type of leukemia, its stage, and the patient's overall health. Common treatment modalities include:

•Chemotherapy: The use of drugs to kill cancer cells or stop their growth.
•Radiation Therapy: High-energy rays are used to target and kill cancer cells.
•Stem Cell Transplant: Healthy stem cells are introduced into the body to replace damaged or cancerous cells.
•Targeted Therapy: Medications that target specific molecules involved in cancer growth.

Prognosis

The prognosis for leukemia varies widely. Advances in treatment have improved outcomes for many people with leukemia, especially in recent years. The outlook depends on factors such as the type of leukemia, the patient's age and overall health, and how well the leukemia responds to treatment.

♦Early detection and prompt, appropriate treatment are crucial in managing leukemia and improving the chances of a positive outcome. Regular follow-up care is often needed to monitor for any signs of recurrence.

Lymphoma

Lymphoma is a type of cancer that originates in the lymphatic system, which is a part of the body's immune system. The lymphatic system includes lymph nodes, lymph vessels, tonsils, spleen, and bone marrow. Lymphomas are characterized by the uncontrolled growth of lymphocytes, a type of white blood cell.

Types of Lymphoma
•Hodgkin Lymphoma (HL):
Hodgkin lymphoma is characterized by the presence of Reed-Sternberg cells, which are large, abnormal lymphocytes. HL is further divided into classical Hodgkin lymphoma and nodular lymphocyte-predominant Hodgkin lymphoma.

•Non-Hodgkin Lymphoma (NHL):
Non-Hodgkin lymphoma includes a diverse group of lymphomas that do not have Reed-Sternberg cells. There are many subtypes of NHL, and they

can be classified as indolent (slow-growing) or aggressive (fast-growing).

Causes and Risk Factors

The exact cause of lymphoma is often unknown, but several risk factors may increase the likelihood of developing the disease:

•Weakened Immune System: Conditions or treatments that suppress the immune system, such as HIV/AIDS or organ transplantation, can increase the risk.
•Age: Lymphoma can occur at any age, but the risk increases with age.
•Family History: Individuals with a family history of lymphoma may have a slightly higher risk.
•Infections: Certain viral and bacterial infections, such as Epstein-Barr virus and Helicobacter pylori, have been associated with an increased risk.

Symptoms

The symptoms of lymphoma can vary depending on the type and stage of the disease but may include:
•Enlarged lymph nodes
•Fatigue
•Unexplained weight loss
•Night sweats
•Fever
•Itching

Diagnosis

Diagnosis involves a combination of medical history, physical examination, blood tests, imaging studies (such as CT or PET scans), and biopsy of affected lymph nodes or other tissues. In Hodgkin lymphoma, the presence of Reed-Sternberg cells is a characteristic feature.

Treatment:
Treatment for lymphoma depends on the type, stage, and overall health of the patient. Common treatment modalities include:

•Chemotherapy: The use of drugs to kill cancer cells or stop their growth.
•Radiation Therapy: High-energy rays are used to target and kill cancer cells.
•Immunotherapy: Boosting the body's immune system to fight cancer.
•Targeted Therapy: Medications that specifically target cancer cells.
•Stem Cell Transplant: Healthy stem cells are introduced into the body to replace damaged or cancerous cells.

Prognosis

The prognosis for lymphoma varies widely, depending on factors such as the type of lymphoma, its stage at diagnosis, and the response to treatment.

Many people with lymphoma respond well to treatment and achieve long-term remission or cure. Regular follow-up care is typically needed to monitor for any signs of recurrence.

♦Early detection and prompt treatment are crucial for improving outcomes in individuals with lymphoma. It's essential for individuals experiencing symptoms or at increased risk to seek medical attention for proper diagnosis and management.

Hemochromatosis

Hemochromatosis is a hereditary disorder characterized by the excessive accumulation of iron in the body. Iron is an essential mineral that plays a crucial role in various physiological processes, including the production of red blood cells. However, when the body absorbs and stores more iron than it needs, it can lead to a condition known as hemochromatosis.

Causes and Types

Hereditary Hemochromatosis (HHC): The most common form of hemochromatosis is hereditary and is caused by a mutation in the HFE gene. This gene regulates the absorption of iron from food in the digestive system. When mutated, it can lead to increased iron absorption.

Secondary Hemochromatosis:This form of hemochromatosis is not primarily caused by genetic factors but may result from other conditions such as excessive blood transfusions, certain types of anemia, or chronic liver disease.

Iron Absorption and Regulation:

In individuals with hemochromatosis, the body tends to absorb more iron from the diet than is needed for normal physiological functions. Over time, this excess iron accumulates in various organs and tissues, including the liver, heart, pancreas, joints, and skin.

Symptoms

Symptoms of hemochromatosis may not appear until middle age or later, as iron gradually builds up in the body over time. Common symptoms include:

•Fatigue
•Joint pain
•Abdominal pain
•Loss of libido
•Heart problems
•Liver dysfunction
•Bronze or grayish skin color

Diagnosis

Diagnosis often involves blood tests to measure serum ferritin levels, transferrin saturation, and total iron-binding capacity. Genetic testing can confirm the presence of the HFE gene mutation associated with hereditary hemochromatosis.

Treatment

The primary treatment for hemochromatosis is phlebotomy, a process similar to blood donation. During phlebotomy, blood is drawn from the patient regularly to reduce the iron levels in the body. This process helps prevent complications associated with excess iron, such as liver damage, diabetes, and heart problems.

In some cases, iron-chelating medications may be used to help remove excess iron from the body. However, phlebotomy remains the most common and effective treatment.

Prognosis

With proper treatment, the prognosis for individuals with hemochromatosis is generally good. Regular monitoring and management of iron levels can prevent or mitigate complications. If diagnosed and treated early, individuals with hemochromatosis can lead normal, healthy lives.

♦It's essential for individuals with a family history of hemochromatosis or those experiencing symptoms to seek medical attention for diagnosis and appropriate management. Early detection and intervention are key to preventing complications associated with excess iron accumulation.

Chapter 8

Musculoskeletal conditions

Musculoskeletal conditions are a broad category of disorders that affect the muscles, bones, joints, tendons, ligaments, and other parts of the musculoskeletal system. The musculoskeletal system provides support, stability, and movement to the body. Conditions affecting this system can have various causes, including injury, inflammation, degeneration, and systemic diseases.

Common musculoskeletal conditions:

Arthritis:

Osteoarthritis: A degenerative joint disease where the protective cartilage that covers the ends of bones wears down over time.

Rheumatoid arthritis: An autoimmune disorder where the immune system attacks the joints, causing inflammation and pain.

Scoliosis:

A sideways curvature of the spine, which can be present at birth or develop during childhood.

Osteoporosis:

A condition characterized by weakened bones, making them more prone to fractures. It often occurs in older individuals, especially postmenopausal women, due to a decrease in bone density.

Gout:

A type of arthritis caused by the buildup of uric acid crystals in the joints, leading to inflammation and pain.

Ankylosing Spondylitis:

A type of inflammatory arthritis that primarily affects the spine, causing pain and stiffness.

Arthritis

Arthritis is a general term that refers to inflammation of the joints. There are more than 100 different types of arthritis, each with its unique characteristics, causes, and treatment approaches. The most common forms of arthritis include *osteoarthritis* and *rheumatoid arthritis.*

Osteoarthritis (OA)

Osteoarthritis is the most prevalent form of arthritis and is often associated with aging. It primarily affects the cartilage, the protective tissue that covers the ends of bones in a joint.

Causes

OA develops when the cartilage gradually breaks down over time. Factors such as aging, joint injury, obesity, and genetic predisposition can contribute to its development.

Symptoms

Common symptoms include joint pain, stiffness, and reduced flexibility. The joints most commonly affected are those in the hands, knees, hips, and spine.

Treatment

Management strategies for osteoarthritis focus on relieving symptoms and improving joint function. This may involve medications (pain relievers, anti-inflammatory drugs), physical therapy, lifestyle changes (weight management, exercise), and in some cases, joint replacement surgery.

Rheumatoid Arthritis (RA)

Rheumatoid arthritis is an autoimmune disorder in which the immune system mistakenly attacks the synovium, the lining of the membranes that surround the joints.

Causes

The exact cause of RA is unknown, but both genetic and environmental factors are believed to contribute. It can affect people of any age.

Symptoms

RA typically causes joint pain, swelling, and stiffness, often affecting joints on both sides of the body simultaneously. It can also lead to systemic symptoms such as fatigue and fever.

Treatment: Treatment for rheumatoid arthritis aims to reduce inflammation, alleviate symptoms, and prevent joint damage. Medications such as disease-modifying antirheumatic drugs (DMARDs), corticosteroids, and nonsteroidal anti-inflammatory drugs (NSAIDs) are commonly prescribed. Physical therapy and lifestyle modifications are also essential components of managing RA.

Other Types of Arthritis:

•**Psoriatic Arthritis**: A form of arthritis that occurs in some individuals with the skin condition psoriasis.

•**Ankylosing Spondylitis:** Primarily affects the spine, causing inflammation and stiffness.

•**Gout**: Caused by the accumulation of uric acid crystals in the joints, leading to sudden and severe attacks of pain, swelling, and redness.

♦It's important to note that early diagnosis and appropriate management are crucial in treating arthritis effectively. A healthcare professional, typically a rheumatologist, can assess symptoms, perform diagnostic tests, and tailor a treatment plan based on the specific type and severity of arthritis. Advances in medical research continue to improve the understanding and treatment options for various forms of arthritis.

Scoliosis

Scoliosis is a medical condition characterized by an abnormal curvature of the spine. Instead of a straight line down the middle of the back, the spine in individuals with scoliosis may curve sideways, resembling an "S" or "C" shape. This condition can affect people of all ages, but it most commonly develops during the growth spurt just before puberty.

Features of Scoliosis
Curvature of the Spine:

The primary characteristic of scoliosis is an abnormal sideways curvature of the spine.

The curvature can occur in different regions of the spine: thoracic (mid-back), lumbar (lower back), or both.

Rotation of the Vertebrae:

In addition to the lateral curvature, there may be some rotation of the vertebrae, causing the ribs on one side of the body to stick out more than on the other side.

Asymmetry in Shoulders, Hips, or Waist:

Scoliosis can lead to uneven shoulders, hips, or waist, as one side of the body may appear higher or more prominent than the other.

Uneven Leg Length:

In some cases, scoliosis may cause a noticeable difference in leg length.

Back Pain and Discomfort:

While many people with scoliosis do not experience pain, some may develop back pain or discomfort, particularly if the curvature is severe.

Causes

•Idiopathic Scoliosis:

The most common form of scoliosis, where the cause is unknown.

Idiopathic scoliosis often develops during adolescence and is more common in females.

•Congenital Scoliosis:

Caused by a defect present at birth in one or more vertebrae, leading to an abnormal curvature as the spine grows.

•Neuromuscular Scoliosis:

Associated with conditions that affect the muscles or nerves, such as cerebral palsy or muscular dystrophy.

•Degenerative Scoliosis:

Develops in adulthood due to the degeneration of the spine's discs and joints.

Diagnosis and Treatment

•Diagnosis: Scoliosis is typically diagnosed through physical examination, X-rays, and, if necessary, other imaging studies.

•Treatment: The approach to treatment depends on the severity of the curvature, the individual's age, and the underlying cause.

•Observation: Mild cases may only require periodic monitoring to ensure that the curvature does not progress.

•Bracing: In some cases, especially for adolescents with moderate curvature, bracing may be recommended to prevent further progression.

•Surgery: Severe cases or those causing significant symptoms may require surgical intervention to straighten and stabilize the spine.

Prognosis

The prognosis for individuals with scoliosis varies depending on factors such as the degree of curvature, age at diagnosis, and the underlying cause.

Most cases of scoliosis do not require surgery and can be effectively managed with conservative measures.

Regular follow-up with healthcare providers, particularly orthopedic specialists, is essential to monitor the progression of scoliosis and determine the most appropriate course of action for each individual. Early detection and intervention are key to optimizing outcomes in managing scoliosis.

Osteoporosis

Osteoporosis is a medical condition characterized by a decrease in bone density and mass, leading to bones that are fragile and more susceptible to fractures. The term "osteoporosis" literally means "porous bones." It is a common condition, particularly in older individuals, and it often progresses silently without symptoms until a fracture occurs. Osteoporosis can affect both men and women, but it is more prevalent in postmenopausal women due to hormonal changes.

Causes and Risk Factors

•Aging: As people age, bone density tends to decrease, and bones may become weaker.

•Hormonal Changes: Postmenopausal women experience a significant decrease in estrogen, a hormone that helps maintain bone density. Men can also experience hormonal changes that contribute to bone loss.

•Genetics: A family history of osteoporosis can increase the risk.

•Nutritional Factors: Inadequate intake of calcium and vitamin D, essential nutrients for bone health, can contribute to osteoporosis.

•Physical Inactivity: Lack of weight-bearing exercise can lead to bone loss.

Certain Medications and Medical Conditions: Long-term use of certain medications, such as glucocorticoids, and certain medical conditions (e.g., rheumatoid arthritis, celiac disease) can increase the risk of osteoporosis.

Symptoms

Osteoporosis is often asymptomatic until a fracture occurs. Common sites for fractures include the hip, spine, and wrist. Fractures in the spine can lead to a loss of height and a stooped or hunched posture.

Diagnosis

•Bone Density Testing: Dual-energy X-ray absorptiometry (DEXA) scans are commonly used to measure bone density and diagnose osteoporosis.

•Medical History and Physical Examination: A healthcare provider will assess risk factors, symptoms, and conduct a physical examination.

Treatment and Management:

•Lifestyle Modifications: Adequate intake of calcium and vitamin D through diet or supplements, weight-bearing exercise, and smoking cessation are essential.

•Medications: Several medications, including bisphosphonates, hormone therapy, and denosumab, may be prescribed to slow down bone loss and reduce fracture risk.

•Fall Prevention: Since fractures are a significant concern, measures to prevent falls, such as improving home safety and balance exercises, are crucial.

♦Osteoporosis is a chronic condition that requires long-term management. Early detection and intervention are essential to prevent fractures and maintain overall bone health. Individuals at risk or diagnosed with osteoporosis should work closely with their healthcare providers to develop a comprehensive plan for prevention and management.

Gout

Gout is a form of inflammatory arthritis characterized by sudden, severe attacks of pain, swelling, redness, and tenderness in the joints, most commonly in the big toe. It occurs when there is an accumulation of uric acid in the blood, leading to the formation of sharp, needle-like crystals in the joints and surrounding tissues.

Features of Gout

Hyperuricemia:

Gout is associated with elevated levels of uric acid in the blood, a condition known as hyperuricemia. Uric acid is a byproduct of the breakdown of purines, which are substances found in certain foods and are also produced by the body.

Acute Attacks (Flares):

Gout typically presents as sudden and intense pain, swelling, and redness in the affected joint, often the big toe. These acute attacks, or flares, can be triggered by factors such as dietary choices, alcohol consumption, dehydration, and certain medications.

Tophi:

Over time, if gout is not adequately managed, uric acid crystals can accumulate in joints, soft tissues, and under the skin, forming lumps called tophi. Tophi can be visible and cause joint deformities.

Chronic Gout:

Some individuals may experience chronic gout, characterized by frequent and prolonged flares, joint damage, and the development of tophi.

Causes and Risk Factors

Diet:

Consuming foods high in purines, such as red meat, organ meats, seafood, and certain alcoholic beverages, can contribute to elevated uric acid levels.

Genetics:

There is a genetic component to gout, and a family history of the condition can increase the risk.

Medical Conditions:

Certain medical conditions, such as kidney disease and metabolic syndrome, can impair the body's ability to excrete uric acid, leading to its accumulation.

Medications:

Some medications, such as diuretics, can increase the risk of gout by reducing the excretion of uric acid.

Diagnosis and Treatment

Diagnosis: A healthcare provider may use blood tests to measure uric acid levels and imaging studies (X-rays or ultrasound) to assess joint damage.

Treatment:

•Medications: Nonsteroidal anti-inflammatory drugs (NSAIDs), colchicine, and corticosteroids are often used to manage acute flares.

•Uric Acid Lowering Medications: Allopurinol and febuxostat are medications that can help lower uric acid levels and prevent future flares.

•Lifestyle Changes: Dietary modifications, reducing alcohol intake, maintaining a healthy weight, and staying hydrated are important in managing gout.

Prevention

Preventive measures include lifestyle modifications, such as adopting a gout-friendly diet and staying well-hydrated.

Long-term management with uric acid-lowering medications may be necessary for those with recurrent or chronic gout.

♦Gout is a chronic condition that requires ongoing management to prevent flares and complications. Individuals with gout should work closely with healthcare providers, including rheumatologists, to develop a comprehensive treatment plan tailored to their specific needs.

Ankylosing

Ankylosing spondylitis (AS) is a type of inflammatory arthritis that primarily affects the spine. It belongs to a group of disorders known as spondyloarthritis, which involves inflammation of the joints and ligaments where the spine and pelvis connect. Ankylosing spondylitis can also impact other joints, as well as organs such as the eyes, heart, and lungs.

Characteristics of Ankylosing Spondylitis:
Inflammation of the Spine:

The hallmark feature of AS is inflammation of the spine, particularly in the sacroiliac joints (the joints that connect the spine to the pelvis).

Over time, the inflammation can lead to fusion of the vertebrae, causing a loss of flexibility and mobility in the spine.

Gradual Onset:

Ankylosing spondylitis often has a gradual onset, with symptoms appearing in late adolescence or early adulthood.

Back Pain and Stiffness:

Persistent and progressive back pain, usually worse in the morning and after periods of inactivity. Stiffness and reduced range of motion in the spine.

Peripheral Joint Involvement:

Besides the spine, AS can affect other joints, such as the hips, shoulders, and knees. Enthesitis:

Inflammation of the entheses, which are the sites where ligaments and tendons attach to bones. This can cause pain and swelling in areas like the heels and bottoms of the feet.

Fatigue:

Many individuals with ankylosing spondylitis experience fatigue, which can be related to both the inflammatory process and the challenges posed by chronic pain and stiffness.

Eye Involvement:

Inflammation of the eyes (uveitis or iritis) is a common extra-articular manifestation of AS.

Causes and Risk Factors

The exact cause of ankylosing spondylitis is not well understood, but it is believed to involve a combination of genetic and environmental factors.

The presence of a specific genetic marker called HLA-B27 is strongly associated with an increased risk of developing AS.

Diagnosis and Treatment

Diagnosis often involves a combination of medical history, physical examination, imaging studies (X-rays, MRI), and blood tests.

Early diagnosis and appropriate management are crucial to prevent complications such as spinal fusion and deformities.

Treatment may include medications to reduce inflammation (NSAIDs, DMARDs), physical therapy, and, in some cases, biologic drugs.

Regular exercise, particularly activities that promote flexibility and posture, is often recommended.

♦Ankylosing spondylitis is a chronic condition that varies in its severity and progression among individuals. Management approaches are typically tailored to the specific needs of each patient, and ongoing care is essential to address symptoms and maintain quality of life. Patients with ankylosing spondylitis often work closely with rheumatologists, who specialize in the treatment of autoimmune and inflammatory conditions.

Gynecological Conditions

Gynecological conditions refer to health issues and disorders that specifically affect the female reproductive system. These conditions can impact various components of the reproductive system, including the uterus, ovaries, fallopian tubes, cervix, and vagina. Gynecological conditions can range from benign and common problems to more serious and potentially life-threatening issues. **Examples of gynecological conditions:**

•Menstrual Disorders:
Dysmenorrhea: Painful menstrual periods.
Menorrhagia: Heavy menstrual bleeding.
Amenorrhea: Absence of menstrual periods.
Endometriosis:
A condition where tissue similar to the lining of the uterus grows outside the uterus, causing pain, inflammation, and the formation of adhesions.

•Vaginitis:
Inflammation or infection of the vagina, often caused by yeast, bacteria, or viruses.

•**Fibroids:**

Noncancerous growths of the uterus that often appear during childbearing years
•**Gynecological Cancers:**
Including ovarian cancer, uterine cancer, cervical cancer, and vulvar cancer

<u>Menstrual disorders</u>

Menstrual disorders encompass a range of conditions that affect the normal menstrual cycle in women. The menstrual cycle is a complex, regulated process involving hormonal changes that prepare the body for a potential pregnancy. Menstrual disorders can disrupt this cycle, leading to irregularities in the timing, duration, or flow of menstrual periods.
 Common types of menstrual disorders:

Dysmenorrhea:
Dysmenorrhea refers to painful menstrual periods. It is one of the most common menstrual disorders and can be classified into two types: primary dysmenorrhea, which is normal menstrual cramps, and secondary dysmenorrhea, which is caused by an underlying reproductive health issue.

Symptoms

Pain in the lower abdomen or pelvis, often accompanied by back pain and headaches.

Menorrhagia:

Menorrhagia involves unusually heavy or prolonged menstrual bleeding. Women with menorrhagia may soak through sanitary pads or tampons quickly, and the bleeding can interfere with daily activities.

Symptoms

Excessive menstrual bleeding, prolonged periods, anemia (due to blood loss).

Amenorrhea:

Amenorrhea is the absence of menstrual periods in women of reproductive age. It can be primary (never having had a period by the age of 16) or secondary (the absence of periods for three or more consecutive cycles in a woman who has previously had regular periods).

Causes

Pregnancy, breastfeeding, hormonal imbalances, stress, excessive exercise, eating disorders, polycystic ovary syndrome (PCOS), and certain medical conditions.

Irregular Menstrual Cycles:

Irregular menstrual cycles involve variations in the length of the menstrual cycle or inconsistent patterns of menstruation.

Causes

Hormonal imbalances, stress, changes in weight, polycystic ovary syndrome (PCOS), thyroid disorders, and certain medications.

Premenstrual Syndrome (PMS):

PMS refers to a combination of physical and emotional symptoms that occur in the days or weeks before menstruation.

Symptoms

Mood swings, irritability, bloating, breast tenderness, fatigue, and changes in appetite.

Treatment for menstrual disorders depends on the underlying cause. It may include lifestyle modifications, hormonal therapy (such as birth control pills), pain relievers, and, in some cases, surgical interventions. Women experiencing persistent or severe menstrual irregularities should consult with a healthcare provider for a thorough evaluation and appropriate management. Regular gynecological check-ups are essential for maintaining reproductive health and addressing menstrual concerns.

<u>Endometriosis</u>

Endometriosis is a chronic medical condition that occurs when tissue similar to the lining of the uterus (endometrium) grows outside the uterus. This tissue, called endometrial implants, may develop on various reproductive organs and structures within the pelvic cavity, such as the ovaries, fallopian tubes, outer surface of the uterus, the pelvic peritoneum (lining of the abdominal cavity), and, in rare cases, other distant organs.

Symptoms

The most common symptom is pelvic pain, which may vary in intensity.
•Painful menstruation (dysmenorrhea).
•Pain during or after sexual intercourse.
Chronic pelvic pain is not necessarily linked to the menstrual cycle.
•Painful bowel movements or urination, especially during menstruation.
•Infertility, though not all women with endometriosis experience fertility issues.

Causes

The exact cause of endometriosis is not fully understood, but several theories exist. Retrograde menstruation, where menstrual blood containing endometrial cells flows backward into the pelvic cavity, is one possible explanation. Other factors like genetic predisposition, immune system dysfunction, and hormonal influences may also contribute.

Diagnosis

Diagnosis often involves a combination of medical history review, pelvic exams, imaging studies (such as ultrasound or MRI), and, in some cases, a surgical procedure called laparoscopy, where a thin tube with a camera is inserted through a small incision to visualize and potentially treat endometriosis.

Treatment

•Pain Management: Over-the-counter pain relievers or prescription medications can help manage pain.

•Hormonal Therapy: Hormonal medications, such as birth control pills, hormonal IUDs, or GnRH agonists, may be prescribed to suppress the menstrual cycle and alleviate symptoms.

•Surgery: In more severe cases or when fertility is a concern, surgical removal of endometriosis implants may be recommended. This can be done through laparoscopic surgery.

Impact on Fertility:

Endometriosis is associated with infertility in some women. The exact relationship between endometriosis and fertility issues is complex and may involve factors such as the location and extent of endometrial implants.

Lifestyle Management

Some lifestyle modifications, such as regular exercise, a balanced diet, and stress management, may help alleviate symptoms.

Endometriosis is a chronic condition that may require long-term management. Treatment approaches are tailored to individual symptoms, the severity of the disease, and the woman's reproductive goals. Early diagnosis and intervention can help manage symptoms and, in some cases, improve fertility outcomes. If someone suspects they have endometriosis or is experiencing symptoms, it's crucial to consult with a healthcare professional for a proper evaluation and personalized treatment plan.

Vaginitis

Vaginitis refers to the inflammation or infection of the vagina, the muscular canal that connects the uterus to the external genitals. This condition is quite common and can result from various causes, including infections, changes in the balance of vaginal bacteria, and irritants. The symptoms and severity of vaginitis can vary depending on the underlying cause.

Causes

•Bacterial Vaginosis (BV): An overgrowth of harmful bacteria in the vagina, disrupting the normal balance of bacteria.

•Yeast Infection (Candidiasis): Overgrowth of the fungus Candida, commonly Candida albicans, in the vagina.

•Trichomoniasis: A sexually transmitted infection caused by the parasite Trichomonas vaginalis.

•Non-infectious causes: These can include allergies or irritants such as certain soaps, bubble baths, douches, or even tight-fitting clothing.

Symptoms

Symptoms can vary depending on the cause but may include:

•Vaginal itching and irritation.

•Abnormal vaginal discharge:

•BV: Thin, grayish-white discharge with a fishy odor.

•Yeast infection: Thick, white, cottage cheese-like discharge.

•Trichomoniasis: Frothy, yellow-green, foul-smelling discharge.

Pain or discomfort during urination or intercourse.

Redness and swelling of the vulva (external genitalia).

Diagnosis

Healthcare providers typically diagnose vaginitis through a combination of medical history, physical examination, and laboratory tests. This may involve examining a sample of vaginal discharge under a microscope, performing a pH test, or using culture or DNA tests to identify specific pathogens.

Treatment

Treatment depends on the underlying cause:
•Bacterial Vaginosis: Antibiotics such as metronidazole or clindamycin.
•Yeast Infection: Antifungal medications, such as fluconazole or topical creams.
•Trichomoniasis: Antiparasitic medications like metronidazole or tinidazole.
•Non-infectious vaginitis: Identifying and avoiding irritants, and sometimes the use of anti-inflammatory medications.

Prevention

Practice good hygiene.
•Avoid douching, as it can disrupt the natural balance of vaginal flora.
•Use mild, unscented soaps and avoid harsh irritants.

•Wear breathable, cotton underwear and avoid tight-fitting pants.
•Practice safe sex to prevent sexually transmitted infections.

♦It's important for individuals experiencing symptoms of vaginitis to seek medical attention for proper diagnosis and treatment. Left untreated, vaginitis can lead to complications and may impact reproductive and sexual health. Healthcare providers can determine the appropriate course of action based on the specific type and cause of vaginitis.

Fibroids

Fibroids, also known as uterine fibroids or leiomyomas, are noncancerous growths of the uterus that often appear during childbearing years. These growths are made up of muscle cells and other tissues that form a mass or lump within or on the walls of the uterus. While fibroids are generally benign, their size and location can lead to various symptoms and complications.

Incidence

Fibroids are quite common, and many women may
have them without experiencing any symptoms.
They are most often diagnosed in women aged 30 to
40.

Types

Fibroids can develop in different parts of the uterus
and can be classified based on their location:
•Intramural: Within the muscular wall of the uterus.
•Submucosal: Protruding into the uterine cavity.
•Subserosal: Projecting to the outside of the uterus.
•Pedunculated: Attached to the uterus by a stalk.

Symptoms

Many women with fibroids are asymptomatic, but
when symptoms do occur, they may include:
•Menstrual changes: Heavier or longer periods,
irregular periods, or spotting between periods.
•Pelvic pain and pressure: Enlarged fibroids or
those pressing on nearby structures can cause
discomfort or a feeling of fullness.
Frequent urination or difficulty emptying the
•bladder: Large fibroids can press against the
bladder.
•Backache or leg pains: Pressure on nerves in the
back due to large fibroids.

Causes

The exact cause of fibroids is unclear, but they are thought to be influenced by hormonal factors, primarily estrogen and progesterone. Genetic factors and family history may also play a role.

Diagnosis

Fibroids are often discovered during a pelvic exam or prenatal ultrasound. Additional imaging studies, such as MRI or ultrasound, may be used to confirm the diagnosis and assess the size and location of the fibroids.

Treatment

Treatment options depend on the severity of symptoms, the size and location of fibroids, and the woman's reproductive goals. Options include:
•Watchful waiting: Monitoring without intervention if the fibroids are small and not causing significant symptoms.
•Medications: Hormonal medications to regulate the menstrual cycle or reduce symptoms.
•Surgery: Surgical options may include myomectomy (removal of fibroids while preserving the uterus) or hysterectomy (removal of the uterus). Uterine artery embolization: A procedure to block the blood supply to the fibroids, causing them to shrink.

♦Although fibroids are frequently seen and generally not dangerous, they have the potential to create substantial discomfort and disrupt a woman's well-being. Women who exhibit symptoms or have worries regarding fibroids should seek advice from a healthcare provider to undergo a thorough assessment and receive direction on the best treatment plan suited to their specific circumstances.

<u>Gynecological cancers</u>

Gynecological cancers are a group of cancers that originate in the female reproductive organs. These cancers can affect various parts of the reproductive system, including the cervix, uterus, ovaries, fallopian tubes, vagina, and vulva. Each type of gynecological cancer has its own characteristics, risk factors, and symptoms. Early detection is crucial for effective treatment and improved outcomes. The main types of gynecological cancers are:

Cervical Cancer:
•Location: Cervix (the lower part of the uterus that connects to the vagina).

•Common Risk Factor: Persistent infection with high-risk strains of human papillomavirus (HPV).
•Screening: Pap smear and HPV testing.
|Symptoms: Abnormal vaginal bleeding, pelvic pain, pain during intercourse.

Uterine (Endometrial) Cancer:

•Location: Uterus (the organ where fetal development occurs during pregnancy).
•Common Risk Factors: Hormonal imbalances, obesity, diabetes, and certain genetic conditions.
•Symptoms: Abnormal vaginal bleeding (especially postmenopausal bleeding), pelvic pain.

Ovarian Cancer:

•Location: Ovaries (the paired organs that produce eggs and hormones).
•Common Risk Factors: Age, family history of ovarian or breast cancer, genetic mutations (e.g., BRCA1, BRCA2).
•Screening: No widely recommended screening test for the general population.
•Symptoms: Vague abdominal discomfort, bloating, pelvic pain, changes in bowel or bladder habits.

Fallopian Tube Cancer:

•Location: Fallopian tubes (tubes that transport eggs from the ovaries to the uterus).

•Risk Factors: Similar to ovarian cancer.

•Symptoms: Often diagnosed at an advanced stage; symptoms may include abdominal pain and swelling.

Vaginal Cancer:

•Location: Vagina (the muscular tube connecting the uterus to the external genitals).

•Risk Factors: Age, history of cervical cancer, HPV infection.

•Symptoms: Abnormal vaginal bleeding, pain during intercourse, pelvic pain.

Vulvar Cancer:

•Location: Vulva (the external genital area).

Risk Factors: Age, chronic vulvar inflammation, HPV infection.

•Symptoms: Itching, pain, tenderness, changes in the color or thickness of the skin.

♦Early detection of gynecological cancers is often challenging because symptoms may be subtle or nonspecific. Regular gynecological exams, screenings, and awareness of potential symptoms are crucial for early diagnosis. Treatment options for gynecological cancers may include surgery, chemotherapy, radiation therapy, hormonal therapy, or a combination of these approaches. The choice of treatment depends on the type and stage of cancer, as well as individual factors such as overall health and preferences. Women should consult with their healthcare providers for personalized cancer screening and prevention plans based on their medical history and risk factors.

Chapter 10
Gastrointestinal (GI) conditions

Gastrointestinal (GI) conditions refer to disorders that affect the digestive system, which includes the organs responsible for processing and absorbing food. The digestive system starts with the mouth and extends to the anus, involving various organs such as the esophagus, stomach, small intestine, large intestine, liver, gallbladder, and pancreas. Gastrointestinal conditions can affect any part of this system and may result from a variety of causes, including infections, inflammation, dietary factors, genetic predisposition, and autoimmune reactions.

Some common gastrointestinal conditions:
Peptic Ulcers: These are open sores that develop on the inner lining of the stomach, upper small intestine, or esophagus. Helicobacter pylori infection or the use of non-steroidal anti-inflammatory drugs (NSAIDs) can contribute to ulcer formation.

Hepatitis: Inflammation of the liver, often caused by viral infections (hepatitis A, B, C, etc.), excessive alcohol consumption, or autoimmune reactions.

Gallstones: Solid particles that form in the gallbladder, typically composed of cholesterol or bilirubin. Gallstones can block the normal flow of bile and lead to pain, inflammation, or infection.

Gastroenteritis: Inflammation of the stomach and intestines, usually caused by viral or bacterial infections. It leads to symptoms such as diarrhea, vomiting, and abdominal cramps.

Gastroesophageal Reflux Disease (GERD): GERD occurs when stomach acid flows back into the esophagus, causing irritation and symptoms such as heartburn. Chronic GERD can lead to complications like esophagitis or Barrett's esophagus.

Peptic ulcer

Peptic ulcers are sores that develop on the inner lining of the stomach, upper small intestine, or the esophagus. These ulcers result from the erosion of the protective lining of these organs, exposing the underlying tissue to stomach acids. The two most common types of peptic ulcers are gastric ulcers, which occur in the stomach, and duodenal ulcers, which develop in the upper part of the small intestine (duodenum).

Causes

•Helicobacter pylori (H. pylori) infection: This bacterium is a major cause of peptic ulcers. It weakens the protective mucous layer of the stomach and duodenum, making it more susceptible to damage from stomach acids.
•Non-steroidal anti-inflammatory drugs (NSAIDs): Regular use of NSAIDs, such as aspirin and ibuprofen, can irritate and erode the lining of the stomach and small intestine, leading to ulcer formation.

Symptoms

•Burning stomach pain: This is the most common symptom and is often felt between the breastbone and the navel.
•Bloating and belching: Especially after meals.
•Nausea and vomiting: Some individuals may experience vomiting that may be bloody.
•Dark, tarry stools: Indicative of bleeding in the digestive tract.

Diagnosi

•Endoscopy: A thin, flexible tube with a camera (endoscope) is used to examine the interior of the digestive tract and identify ulcers.

•Upper gastrointestinal (GI) series: X-rays are taken after drinking a contrast solution to visualize the stomach and duodenum.

H. pylori testing: Blood, stool, or breath tests can determine the presence of H. pylori.

Treatment

•Antibiotics: If H. pylori infection is present, a course of antibiotics is prescribed to eliminate the bacteria.

•Proton pump inhibitors (PPIs) and H2 blockers: These medications reduce stomach acid production, promoting ulcer healing.

•Antacids: Provide quick relief by neutralizing stomach acid.

•Cytoprotective agents: Medications that enhance the protective lining of the stomach.

Complications

•Bleeding ulcers: The erosion of blood vessels within the ulcer can lead to bleeding, resulting in symptoms like black, tarry stools or vomiting blood. Perforation: In rare cases, ulcers can create a hole in the wall of the stomach or intestine, causing a life-threatening condition requiring immediate medical attention.

Prevention

•H. pylori eradication: Taking precautions to avoid H. pylori infection, such as practicing good hygiene.
•Limiting NSAID use: Using NSAIDs cautiously, especially in individuals with a history of ulcers.
♦It's essential to consult a healthcare professional if one suspects the presence of a peptic ulcer or experiences symptoms like persistent stomach pain, nausea, or vomiting blood. Early diagnosis and appropriate treatment can prevent complications and promote healing.

Hepatitis

Hepatitis is an inflammation of the liver, typically caused by viral infections, although it can also result from exposure to certain medications, toxins, or autoimmune diseases. The severity and duration of hepatitis can vary widely, ranging from a mild illness to a serious, lifelong condition.

There are several types of viral hepatitis, including hepatitis A, hepatitis B, hepatitis C, hepatitis D, and hepatitis E.

Viral Types:

•Hepatitis A (HAV): Usually transmitted through contaminated food or water. It is a short-term infection, and most people recover fully with no lasting liver damage.

•Hepatitis B (HBV): Transmitted through contact with infected blood, body fluids, or from an infected mother to her newborn during childbirth. It can be acute (short-term) or chronic (long-term).

•Hepatitis C (HCV): Mainly spread through blood-to-blood contact, often through the sharing of needles or other drug injection equipment. It can also be chronic and lead to long-term liver problems.

•Hepatitis D (HDV): A unique type that can only infect individuals who are already infected with hepatitis B. It can lead to severe illness.

•Hepatitis E (HEV): Usually transmitted through contaminated water. It is similar to hepatitis A and is typically acute.

Non-Viral Causes:

•Alcoholic hepatitis: Excessive alcohol consumption can cause inflammation and damage to the liver.

•Toxic hepatitis: Exposure to certain chemicals, drugs, or toxins can lead to liver inflammation.

•Autoimmune hepatitis: The immune system mistakenly attacks the liver cells, leading to inflammation.

Symptoms

•Common symptoms: Fatigue, nausea, vomiting, abdominal pain, and jaundice (yellowing of the skin and eyes).

•Chronic hepatitis: Some individuals with viral hepatitis may not experience symptoms for years, even though the virus is gradually causing liver damage.

Diagnosis

•Blood tests: These can detect the presence of viral particles, antibodies, and assess liver function.

•Imaging studies: Such as ultrasound or CT scans may be used to evaluate the liver's condition.

Treatment

Antiviral medications: Some forms of viral hepatitis have specific antiviral drugs.

Supportive care: Rest, proper nutrition, and avoiding substances that can further damage the liver are important.

Prevention

•Vaccination: Vaccines are available for hepatitis A and hepatitis B, providing effective prevention.

•Safe practices: Avoiding risky behaviors such as unprotected sex, sharing needles, and practicing good hygiene can reduce the risk of hepatitis.

Complications

•Cirrhosis: Chronic hepatitis can lead to the scarring of the liver, reducing its function.
•Liver cancer: Long-term inflammation increases the risk of liver cancer.
•Liver failure: In severe cases, hepatitis can lead to liver failure, a life-threatening condition.

♦Prompt diagnosis and appropriate medical care are crucial for managing hepatitis, especially chronic forms of the disease. Early intervention can help prevent complications and improve outcomes. If you suspect you have hepatitis or are at risk, consult a healthcare professional for evaluation and guidance.

Gallstones

Gallstones are solid particles that form in the gallbladder, a small organ beneath the liver. The gallbladder plays a role in the digestion process by storing and releasing bile, a digestive fluid produced by the liver. Gallstones can develop when the balance of substances that make up bile—such as cholesterol, bilirubin, and calcium—is disrupted, leading to the formation of solid particles.

Types of Gallstones

•Cholesterol stones: These are the most common type and are primarily composed of cholesterol. Imbalances in bile components can cause cholesterol to crystallize and form stones.
•Pigment stones: These are less common and are made of bilirubin, a yellow-brown pigment that forms when red blood cells are broken down. They can occur when the liver produces too much bilirubin or when the gallbladder doesn't effectively empty.

Risk Factors

•Gender: Women are more likely to develop gallstones than men.
Age: Gallstones are more common in older adults.
•Obesity: Excess body weight, especially rapid weight loss, increases the risk.
•Pregnancy: The hormonal changes during pregnancy can contribute to gallstone formation.
Certain diseases and conditions: Conditions such as cirrhosis, diabetes, and certain blood disorders can increase the risk.

Symptoms

•Most gallstones are asymptomatic: Many people with gallstones don't experience symptoms and may not even be aware of their presence.

•Symptomatic gallstones: When gallstones cause symptoms, the most common is biliary colic—an intense pain in the upper abdomen that may radiate to the back or shoulder. Pain often occurs after meals, particularly those high in fat.

Complications

•Cholecystitis: Inflammation of the gallbladder, often occurring when a gallstone blocks the cystic duct.

•Pancreatitis: Gallstones can block the pancreatic duct, leading to inflammation of the pancreas.

•Gallbladder obstruction: A stone can obstruct the bile duct, causing jaundice, abdominal pain, and potentially serious complications.

Diagnosis

•Ultrasound: The most common imaging test for diagnosing gallstones.

•Blood tests: These can identify signs of inflammation or infection in the gallbladder or pancreas.

Treatment

•Watchful waiting: Asymptomatic gallstones may not require treatment.

•Medications: Ursodeoxycholic acid may be prescribed to dissolve cholesterol stones.

•Surgery: Cholecystectomy, the removal of the gallbladder, is a common and effective treatment for symptomatic gallstones. Laparoscopic surgery is a minimally invasive approach.

•Endoscopic procedures: In some cases, gallstones can be removed using endoscopic techniques.
Prevention:

•Maintaining a healthy weight: Avoiding rapid weight loss and adopting a balanced diet.

•Eating a high-fiber diet: A diet rich in fruits, vegetables, and whole grains may help prevent gallstones.

♦If someone experiences symptoms of gallstones, such as severe abdominal pain, it's crucial to seek medical attention for proper diagnosis and treatment. Gallstone complications can be serious, and early intervention is important to prevent complications.

Gastroenteritis is an inflammation of the gastrointestinal tract, which includes the stomach and the intestines. This condition is commonly referred to as the stomach flu or stomach bug, although it is not caused by the influenza virus.

Gastroenteritis

Gastroenteritis is typically caused by viral or bacterial infections, although parasites and certain toxins can also be responsible. It is a common condition that can affect people of all ages.

Causes

•Viral gastroenteritis: Common viruses causing gastroenteritis include norovirus, rotavirus, adenovirus, and astrovirus. Norovirus, in particular, is a frequent cause of outbreaks in settings like cruise ships and healthcare facilities.
•Bacterial gastroenteritis: Bacteria such as Salmonella, Escherichia coli (E. coli), Campylobacter, and Shigella can cause gastroenteritis. Contaminated food or water is a common source of bacterial infections.
•Parasitic gastroenteritis: Parasites like Giardia lamblia and Cryptosporidium can cause gastroenteritis, often through contaminated water.

Symptoms

•Diarrhea: Often watery and frequent.

•Nausea and vomiting: Common symptoms, especially in viral infections.

•Abdominal cramps: Pain or discomfort in the stomach area.

•Fever: May accompany viral or bacterial infections.

Transmission

•Person-to-person: Viral gastroenteritis is highly contagious and can spread through direct contact with an infected person or by touching surfaces or objects contaminated with the virus.

•Contaminated food and water: Bacterial and parasitic gastroenteritis often result from consuming contaminated food or water.

Diagnosis:

•Clinical evaluation: Healthcare providers typically diagnose gastroenteritis based on symptoms and a physical examination.

•Stool tests: In some cases, a stool sample may be analyzed to identify the specific cause, especially if the symptoms are severe or prolonged.

Treatment:

•Hydration: Maintaining fluid intake is crucial to prevent dehydration, especially in cases of diarrhea and vomiting.

Dietary adjustments: Gradually reintroducing bland foods after symptoms improve.

•Medications: In some cases, antiemetics (for nausea) or antidiarrheal medications may be recommended. However, these are generally not advised for certain types of infections.

Prevention

•Hand hygiene: Regular handwashing is essential, especially after using the bathroom and before handling food.

•Safe food handling: Proper food storage, preparation, and cooking can help prevent bacterial and parasitic infections.

•Vaccination: Vaccines are available for certain causes of gastroenteritis, such as the rotavirus vaccine for children.

Duration

•Acute: Gastroenteritis is typically acute and self-limiting, with symptoms resolving within a few days to a week. However, some cases may persist longer, especially if caused by certain parasites.

♦While most cases of gastroenteritis resolve on their own, it's important to seek medical attention if symptoms are severe, persistent, or if there are signs of dehydration. Infants, elderly individuals, and people with weakened immune systems may be more susceptible to complications and may require more careful monitoring and medical care.

Gastroesophageal Reflux Disease (GERD)

Gastroesophageal Reflux Disease, commonly known as GERD, is a chronic digestive disorder that occurs when stomach acid or, occasionally, stomach content, flows back into the esophagus. The esophagus is the tube that carries food from the mouth to the stomach. The backward flow of acid can irritate the lining of the esophagus, leading to various symptoms and potential complications.

Causes

The lower esophageal sphincter (LES) is a ring of muscle that acts as a valve between the esophagus and the stomach. In individuals with GERD, this valve may weaken or relax abnormally, allowing stomach acid to flow back into the esophagus.

Factors contributing to GERD include **obesity, pregnancy, hiatal hernia, smoking, and certain dietary habits.**

Symptoms

Common symptoms of GERD include:

•Heartburn: A burning sensation in the chest or throat.
•Regurgitation: Sour or bitter-tasting acid backing up into the throat or mouth.
•Dysphagia: Difficulty swallowing.
•Chest pain: May be mistaken for a heart attack.

Complications

If left untreated, GERD can lead to complications such as:

•Esophagitis: Inflammation of the esophagus.
•Barrett's esophagus: Changes in the lining of the esophagus that can increase the risk of esophageal cancer.
•Strictures: Narrowing of the esophagus due to scar tissue formation.
•Respiratory problems: Stomach acid can be aspirated into the lungs, leading to issues such as asthma, chronic cough, or pneumonia.

•Diagnosis: Diagnosis is often based on a combination of symptoms, medical history, and sometimes diagnostic tests. Tests may include upper endoscopy, esophageal pH monitoring, and imaging studies.

Treatment

Treatment strategies for GERD aim to alleviate symptoms, promote healing of the esophagus, and prevent complications. Common approaches include:

•Lifestyle modifications: Such as weight loss, avoiding trigger foods (spicy, fatty, acidic), and raising the head of the bed.
•Medications: Antacids, H2 blockers, and proton pump inhibitors (PPIs) can reduce acid production or neutralize existing acid.
•Surgery: In severe cases, when medications and lifestyle changes are not effective, surgical procedures like fundoplication may be considered.

Prevention

Adopting healthy lifestyle habits can help prevent or manage GERD. This includes maintaining a healthy weight, avoiding large meals before bedtime, quitting smoking, and managing stress.

♦It's important for individuals experiencing symptoms of GERD to seek medical attention, as chronic acid reflux can lead to serious complications. A healthcare provider can help determine the most appropriate course of treatment based on the severity of symptoms and individual health factors.